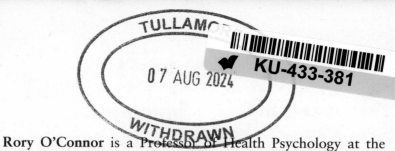
**Rory O'Connor** is a Professor of Health Psychology at the University of Glasgow where he leads the Suicidal Behaviour Research Laboratory. He is a world leader on suicide research and prevention and has been working in this area for 25 years. In January 2021, Rory became President of the International Association for Suicide Prevention (IASP) and he is also a past President of the International Academy of Suicide Research (IASR). He has published extensively in the field of suicide and self-harm and has contributed to six BBC documentaries on suicide, including *Suicide and Me* with the rapper Professor Green and *Our Silent Emergency* with Roman Kemp. You can find him on Twitter: @suicideresearch

*To all those who have lost a loved one to suicide*
*and to those who struggle daily to stay alive*

# When It Is Darkest

## Why people die by suicide and what we can do to prevent it

RORY O'CONNOR

**Vermilion**
LONDON

1

Vermilion, an imprint of Ebury Publishing,
20 Vauxhall Bridge Road,
London SW1V 2SA

Vermilion is part of the Penguin Random House group of companies
whose addresses can be found at global.penguinrandomhouse.com

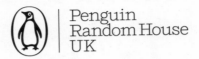

Copyright © Rory O'Connor 2021

Rory O'Connor has asserted his right to be identified as the author of this
Work in accordance with the Copyright, Designs and Patents Act 1988

First published in Great Britain in 2021 by Vermilion

www.penguin.co.uk

A CIP catalogue record for this book is available from the British Library

ISBN 9781785043437

Printed and bound in Great Britain by Clays Ltd, Elcograf S.p.A.

The authorised representative in the EEA is Penguin Random House
Ireland, Morrison Chambers, 32 Nassau Street, Dublin D02 YH68.

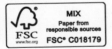

Penguin Random House is committed to a
sustainable future for our business, our readers
and our planet. This book is made from Forest
Stewardship Council® certified paper.

The information in this book has been compiled by way of general
guidance in relation to the specific subjects addressed. It is not a
substitute and not to be relied on for medical, healthcare, pharmaceutical
or other professional advice on specific circumstances and in specific
locations. Please consult your GP before changing, stopping or starting
any medical treatment. So far as the author is aware the information
given is correct and up to date as at December 2020. Practice, laws and
regulations all change, and the reader should obtain up to date
professional advice on any such issues. All names and identifying
characteristics of the individuals mentioned in this book have been
changed to protect their privacy. The author and publishers disclaim,
as far as the law allows, any liability arising directly or indirectly from
the use, or misuse, of the information contained in this book.

# Contents

# Introduction

'YOU'RE NOT GOING to kill yourself, are you?'

That was one of the first things that my mother said to me, 25 years ago, when I embarked on a PhD on suicide. She was concerned about the emotional toll that working in the field of suicide research would have on me and would regularly check in to make sure that I was looking after my own mental health.

'Of course not,' I replied.

'Are you sure?' she pushed, seeking further confirmation.

To be honest, I didn't know how to answer her question. It wasn't something that I had really thought about. As a 21-year-old, I felt indestructible and had never really invested much time in looking after my own mental health. Also, I had no direct experience of suicide at that stage. I had always been intrigued by mental health, although my decision to study suicide wasn't planned; it was serendipitous. As an undergraduate psychology student at Queen's University Belfast, I had been researching depression and I had intended to continue this work into my PhD.

However, in the summer of 1994, just after my graduation, out of the blue, one of my professors, Noel, telephoned me, asking whether I'd be interested in doing a PhD on suicide. I jumped at the chance. When I thought about it, it was the obvious next step for me. Suicide is the most shocking outcome from depression and, although the suicide rates among young men across the UK in the early nineties were on the increase, there had been little relevant research in Northern Ireland. That day, when I agreed, I couldn't quite envisage what a PhD on suicide would look like, but I grabbed the opportunity with both hands and just ran with it. And there it began – suicide research was to become my life's passion. Little did I know, though, that many years later Noel would lose his own mental health fight by his own hand. I often think about him reaching out to me, it was like my *Sliding Doors* moment; although I'll never know for certain, I doubt I would have become a suicide researcher without him, I think my life would have taken a very different path. For this I am eternally grateful. To this day I wake up every morning with as much drive and enthusiasm (if not more) to make a difference as I did in my twenties. Perhaps I should have reached out to Noel in his hour of need. I really wish I had. I'll always regret that I didn't do more for him. Guilt and regret are such commons emotions after a suicide.

Returning to my mother's question, I hadn't anticipated the emotional toll of doing a PhD that involved interviewing people who had attempted suicide and learning, at first hand, the intimate details of those who had died by suicide. I don't know why, it was obvious. Of course it would be draining. To this day, I vividly remember the first person I interviewed as part of my PhD: Greg, a man in his forties who had been admitted to hospital after a suicide attempt. He had taken a massive overdose hours before. He was lucky to be alive, but he seemed so angry when I clapped eyes on him from across the ward. Although I had role-played in advance what I might say, I was still petrified as I approached his hospital bed. I was starting to sweat, hoping I wouldn't say the wrong thing.

'Hello, I am a psychologist who is carrying out research and I'd like to ask you some questions about what happened last night. Is that okay?' I enquired. I expected him to say no, but to my surprise, and as I would learn, like most patients who I approached following a suicide attempt, he agreed.

We talked about his life, his mental health, his recent long-term relationship breakdown, his distant past and how he came to attempt suicide the night before. He wanted to be heard. Although he was older than me, he was no different from me – no different from any one of us; he was someone going through a bad patch, struggling to get through each day. Also, I had misjudged him; he wasn't angry, but despondent – he was stuck, trapped, feeling a burden to loved ones. When I asked how he felt now, after his suicide attempt, and whether anything had changed for him, he told me, tearfully: 'No, nothing has changed. I don't care. I feel the same way as I did last night. I feel as depressed and as useless as I did yesterday.' And he was right, nothing had changed – his relationship was still broken and he was no closer to getting the support for the trauma he had experienced as a child. He had been diagnosed with an adjustment disorder and would soon be discharged, receiving no more support beyond a letter sent to his GP. I felt so helpless; it was my first experience of the emotional impact of seeing someone in such acute distress but not being able to help. He was leaving hospital with more problems than when he had arrived barely conscious in an ambulance hours earlier. Now he had to face his family.

'They're ashamed of me, they think I am so bloody selfish. How could I do this to them?' he said at one point. There wasn't much I could say in response. At the end of the interview, he thanked me, and, while I was wondering why, as if reading my mind, he added, 'thanks for listening'.

I learned so many valuable lessons that day and in those early days in the observational ward linked to the emergency department at Belfast's City Hospital. I learned about the importance of listening and the power of silence. I learned about the potency of my own fears as well as the pain of suicidal distress. I learned the value of being alongside someone in their own distress and the shame so often linked to suicide. I knew then that I had made the right decision that summer and I resolved to do whatever I could, no matter how small, to tackle suicide.

Still, my mother's words have stayed with me; with others – my wife, family, friends and colleagues – now adding to the self-care chorus. And, ever since then, I've been having the *will-I-die-by-suicide* conversations with myself intermittently, usually when grappling with sleep or if I have been working late at night, or when something is really troubling me. It's as if they just sneak up on me. They've also become much more frequent in my forties, waxing and waning, coming and going with the ups and downs of life. Even when I am not having the 'will I, won't I' conversation, never a day passes when I don't think about suicide, its causes or consequences. I live, breathe and, quite literally, dream about suicide.

It is not that I have ever been acutely suicidal, but since the mid- to late nineties, I've spent all of my working life studying suicide; trying to get inside the mind of someone who is suicidal and striving to understand the complex set of factors that leads to suicide. I am a Professor of Health Psychology at the University of Glasgow where I direct the Suicidal Behaviour Research Laboratory, a research group dedicated to understanding and preventing suicide. In addition to my research at the university, I work with many national and international organisations tasked with preventing suicide. I also travel up and down the country delivering talks about suicide to the general public. This is easily one of the most rewarding aspects of my job, seeing first-hand how our research is helping others understand their own or their loved one's distress. It is so important that scientists communicate their research findings as widely as possible, especially when they genuinely relate to issues of life and death. In the course of my work, I am privileged to talk to people who have been bereaved by suicide and to those who struggle to stay alive, as well as to those who have recovered from suicidal crises. I am continually humbled by the trust people place in me and my research team when they share their most private life stories.

Late one night, while on a recent holiday with my family in Crete, I experienced the *will-I-die-by-suicide* thoughts again. I might add that this is no reflection on the holiday, which was idyllic – 30-degree heat, turquoise sea and copious amounts of food and drink, and great company. Such holidays feel like a distant memory now as I write this in the midst of the COVID-19 pandemic. I think it was the combination of the humidity, difficulty unwinding from work (my summer holiday is the only time of the year when I turn off my email) and Catholic guilt, which takes hold when I am not working. That night and for the previous few weeks, this goddam book, yes, this one, had rarely been far from my waking and nocturnal mind. For several years I had wanted to write a book on suicide for the general public, to reach those who do not read scientific papers. Something that would speak to those who have lost loved ones to suicide, who have been suicidal or work with people in crisis, as well as the wider public trying to understand this complex phenomenon. Also, I wanted the book to be personal, to convey something of my own experiences, but I was concerned, as a private person, about giving away too much about myself. I suppose I was paralysed by self-disclosure anxiety. As someone who has spent all of my adult life endeavouring to portray myself as competent and self-assured, I kept asking myself why on earth I would risk exposing any vulnerabilities, uncertainties and neuroses in a book. After many attempts, I just couldn't settle on a way forward.

I had a breakthrough though, at around 4am that night on holiday, unable to sleep, just focusing on the whirr of the air conditioning and trying to silence my mind. As had happened so often in the past, the *will-I-die-by-suicide* thoughts surfaced one by one, though, this time, they were pretty intrusive: 'Will I die by suicide?', 'Could I kill myself?, 'Am I frightened of dying?' . . . But what was different that night was that for the first time I stayed with the thoughts, trying to make sense of them, asking myself, 'What do they mean?', 'Why do they keep coming back?', 'What's wrong with me?'. In the past I'd bat them away as soon as they entered my conscious awareness, finding them uncomfortable and disconcerting. I pondered whether it was my immersion in suicide research that triggered such thoughts, or whether it was because, with almost every passing year, someone else I know dies by suicide and I cannot help but compare myself to them. My reasoning continued: 'Surely, therefore, it isn't surprising that I am preoccupied with my own vulnerability and possible suicide?' What is more, since the age of 23, when my father died suddenly of a heart attack at 51, I've been fixated on my own mortality. I wondered whether I was unconsciously planning my own death, but by suicide rather than a heart attack. Also, I considered the fact that I'd been having these thoughts much more frequently recently, which coincided with my own personal discontent with life, agitation and general malaise in the past few years. Indeed this triumvirate, which has marred much of my forties, led me to start personal therapy five years ago.

Unexpectedly, though, the puzzling over my own thoughts of suicide led to a sea change in my thinking that night; confronting them allowed me to acknowledge and accept that it was okay to have such thoughts. This step forward also had echoes of what happened to me a few years earlier when I started therapy. At the age of 42, for the first time in my adult life, I had reached out for help because I was struggling to cope. I was incredibly unhappy, perhaps depressed, but I couldn't understand why. Thankfully, undertaking weekly psychodynamic psychotherapy helped me immensely and still does. Initially, it was upsetting and disconcerting. I felt extremely exposed and vulnerable. As a result, I kept my visits secret, telling only those closest to me. I have come a long way since my first session in May 2016. I've a better understanding of who I am, I'm more accepting of my own flaws and I'm definitely happier, much, much happier. It has also helped me professionally. It has given me a deeper appreciation of the darkness of despair, the nothingness of living and the unbearable loneliness even when surrounded by others.

Without doubt, therapy has been a turning point for me and for my mental health. For most of my adult life, I'd been so driven by making my career a success that I'd largely ignored my emotional and mental health needs. I was the upbeat extrovert, always positive while concealing, for the most part, my nail-biting neuroses. I had to do everything at a million miles per hour. Metaphorically, I'd be running as fast as I could from one thing to another. I didn't make the time or space to nourish my own mental health. The irony isn't lost on me, given the focus of my working life!

I remember an early session with my therapist, when she asked whether my constant running represented me running away from something. We also explored whether I feared that if I slowed down, then I might have to deal with my own discontent and emptiness. Or was it the death of my father? I've spent the last few years trying to make sense of this. I think that, initially, my efforts to cram in everything were driven by my preoccupation with dying young. But latterly I believe that my fear of slowing down was because I didn't want to confront my own emotional needs. This is reflected in a diary entry I made not long after starting therapy:

> It is so easy to burst my 'externally-facing' confidence and self-esteem. In therapy recently, I talked about how, sometimes, when I am ruminating heavily, I'll try to picture myself in a box – and for some reason that gives me some comfort and assumed protection. I wish I wasn't so psychologically thin-skinned, if I just keep going, then the rumination will be blocked out and I'll be able to relax.

One of the reasons I am disclosing my own struggles here is because reaching out for help has been transformative for me. So I hope that my experience will encourage others to consider doing the same, especially if they are reticent. Although I still have regular battles with myself and my mental health, I have found a way that works for me that is much more healthy and manageable. Also, the idea of psychological thin skins is something I return to later as I explore the factors that can lead to suicide.

Returning to that night in Crete when I had the break-through: it was as if something inside me had been unlocked, a eureka moment of sorts. The thoughts were no longer disturbing, but oddly comforting; it was like a weight lifting. Then, with the sun rising, my thoughts returned to this book; after being stuck for so long I could now see a way forward. I was able to visualise a structure that was personal as well as focused on understanding the complexity of suicide and communicating the latest research evidence about what can be done to alleviate the risk of suicide. I don't know what triggered the change that night. Perhaps being on holiday allowed me the time and space to think about my own vulner-abilities without the never-ending intrusion of work. Perhaps it was the result of the safe space of having undergone several years of therapy. Whatever it was, the next morning, after a fitful few hours' sleep, I wrote the first few hundred words of this book.

Before finally falling off to sleep that night – or, more accur-ately, early that morning – my thoughts drifted to the day I was first touched personally by suicide, when I received the news that one of my closest friends, Clare, had died.

I was in my office when I took the call on my mobile.

'She's gone, Clare's gone,' Dave said.

'What do you mean?' I couldn't understand.

It was an unexpected call. Dave and Clare were living in Paris, it was the middle of the day and we usually planned calls in advance. Why was he phoning? I had been speaking to them both a few weeks before and had been in email contact with Clare recently. I was looking forward to their return to Scot-land. Clare had a lectureship at a university in Scotland, but they had been living in Paris for the past year, as Dave had a fellowship and Clare had used sabbatical leave to spend a lot of time there that year. She, they, adored Paris.

I remember standing up, confused, quickly pacing up and down my narrow room. I might have asked again, what on earth did he mean that 'Clare's gone'?

'Clare's dead,' Dave replied. I still didn't, couldn't, understand. Not even for a split second did I think Dave was going to tell me that Clare was dead.

Much of the rest of the conversation is a haze to me. I was in shock. I just couldn't take it in. I still couldn't understand what Dave meant. 'Clare's dead.' Does he not mean that she's gone away somewhere? What did he mean, 'Clare's dead'? Through tears, Dave told me what had happened: Clare had killed herself. I was devastated. While Dave was talking, my inner voice kept repeating over and over again, 'Clare's dead, Clare's dead', each time getting louder and louder.

That was September 2008. Clare was 40 and I was 35. We had met many years before when we were both PhD students in Belfast and had been friends ever since. The next day, when I flew to Paris to be with Dave, I still couldn't believe that Clare was no longer with us. Everywhere we went, I kept expecting to see her. None of it made any sense. For months after her death, Clare would appear in my dreams, always telling me she was okay and not to worry.

I remain devastated by Clare's death. It changed me as a person. Apart from the personal loss of losing such an amazing friend, it made me question my professional life. My immediate reaction was that I had failed Clare, Dave and her family. That I was a complete failure. Initially, I didn't know whether I would be able to continue working in suicide research – I found it really difficult because everything I did was a reminder of Clare. But I am so glad that I did stick with it. It is this sense of failure that continues to drive me academically, striving to better understand the factors that lead to suicide and to develop new ways to keep the most vulnerable safe. Clare still comes up in my weekly therapy sessions. I cry less now about her death, but I still do. Her influence is still so pervasive in my life. It serves as a daily reminder of my own fragility, of all our fragilities.

Every one of us has our own experience, either directly or indirectly, of suicide. It is a public health crisis that affects millions of people each year across the world. Every one of us will know someone who has died by suicide or we will know someone who has been affected by suicide, or both. Sadly though, for the most part, we are reluctant to talk about suicide and frightened to ask someone whether they are suicidal or not. This has to change. It is crucial that we promote the conversations around suicide, so that more people will feel less alone and get the help and support that they require.

Suicide is one of the last remaining taboos. It is 'the big S', because some people are still reluctant to utter its name. It reminds me of the taboo around cancer 20 or 30 years ago, when it was frequently referred to as 'the big C'. Sadly, suicide and talking about suicide are plagued by stigma, myth and misunderstanding. In this book, my aim is to get to the heart of this most tragic of human outcomes, challenging myths and misunderstandings. I also aim to illustrate the vulnerabilities in all of us, but crucially to show how these vulnerabilities can be catalysts to make us stronger. I will take you through the research evidence and the different ways in which we try to understand suicide, but importantly I will also provide a voice for those who are suicidal or who have been bereaved by suicide. I have deliberately steered away from adopting a text-book approach to writing this book. As suicide can affect anyone, I want it to be accessible to as wide a readership as possible. There are other books that provide the precise details about every single approach to understanding and preventing suicide. This book is not a checklist of every risk factor or suicide prevention strategy. That is not its purpose.

Rather, I have tried to do something different with *When It Is Darkest*. I have combined the personal with the professional – by telling something of people's stories, including my own, I have tried to convey a sense of what I have learned from my life and from my research into this most devastating of phenomena. This is my journey through research into suicide, including how suicide has touched me personally. In this book, I try to make sense of suicide by drawing from the experiences of people I've met and in so doing I'll share the stories of those who have been suicidal and those who have lost loved ones to suicide. In all instances, I have changed personal details about their lives or what happened to them to preserve their anonymity. I have combined different encounters into a single description, but, although I have changed some details, the message is unaltered and is true to the encounter. I have learned so much from the countless people who have been part of my journey so far in suicide research and prevention, and for this I am truly grateful.

I will introduce some of the common reasons why people die by suicide and the factors associated with suicide. I will try to make sense of suicidal thoughts and why, for some, they result in suicide attempts and in others they end in death. Contrary to some media reports, suicide is not caused by a single factor. Instead, it is the end product of a complex set of biological, psychological, clinical, social and cultural determinants that come together in a perfect storm. For most, suicide is not about wanting to end one's life but about wanting unbearable mental pain to end. Throughout the book, I will untangle the factors that lead to the emergence of this pain by taking you through some of the key determinants of suicide.

If you have been affected by suicide, especially if you have lost a loved one, reading this book may give rise to difficult and painful emotions. Self-care is so important, so please look after yourself. I've included details of some organisations at the back of the book that may be helpful if you need support (see page 277).

Finally, if you have ever been suicidal, have lost someone to suicide or are supporting someone who is suicidal or self-harming, my biggest hope is that this book helps, in some small way, in making sense of your own pain or the pain of those who struggle or have lost the battle to live.

# Part 1

# Suicide: An Overview

One person dies by suicide every 40 seconds somewhere in the world.[1] Every death by suicide is an unbearable personal tragedy and the ripples of suicide are vast, stretching well beyond our immediate families. Too many children lose parents, countless partners are left behind, friends and colleagues are devastated; schools, workplaces and communities are stunned by loss each and every day. For a long time, it was suggested that for every person who dies by suicide six people will be potentially directly affected by their death. However, this number has been shown to be a gross underestimate. In 2018, an American study, which spawned the hashtag #notsix on social media, led by clinical psychologist Julie Cerel, showed that 135 people will know each person who dies by suicide.[2] Although this number includes more distant social acquaintances, many of whom will not be directly bereaved, as well as the very closest of contacts, it still highlights the vast reach of suicide. The impact of each suicide is akin to a social bomb exploding, with the extent of the devastation impossible to predict.

The first time I was exposed to suicide was in the early nineties when I was a fresher at university, and a classmate lost their cousin to suicide. The cousin had celebrated his twenty-first birthday a month before and on the night of his death he had been out social-ising, seemingly in good spirits. But he went home later that evening and took his own life, not long after saying goodnight to his friends. I remember being puzzled by his death as it appeared to come out of the blue, but I didn't give it much thought at the time. Sadly, his death was not unusual in Northern Ireland at that time when suicides by young men were on the increase.[3] Although I was not directly bereaved on that occasion, I was affected vicari-ously, feeling some of the pain that my friend went through. That was one death in one family in one country. Worldwide, the World Health Organization (WHO) tells us that at least 800,000 people die by suicide each year.[4] This translates to as many as 108 million people newly exposed to suicide annually. That's more than one and a half times the population of the UK or a third of the popula-tion of the USA.

Those left behind are overwhelmed by *what ifs* and *if onlys*, often being at a loss to understand why their loved one took their own life. However, before addressing why so many people die by their own hand, I will briefly take you through who is at risk of sui-cide and when. I will also outline some of the challenges we face as we try to get to grips with this most baffling of phenomena. In Chapter 2, we will hear from those who have been directly affected by suicide, which will provide a direct insight into what suicidal pain feels like. Finally, in Chapter 3 I will describe many of the com-mon myths around suicide and explain how they developed and what more needs to be done to ensure that they are dispelled.

# 1

# The How, Who and When of Suicide

LET'S START WITH the term suicide and the challenges of determining that someone took their own life. In almost all countries of the world we use the word suicide to describe a self-inflicted death; this is straightforward and not controversial. However, how do we determine that a person intended to end their life rather than their death being accidental? This is easier if a suicide note is found saying that the deceased had intended to take their own life. However, less than one third of people who die by suicide leave a suicide note, so in the majority of cases we don't have any direct evidence.[1] I also know of instances where, despite a suicide note being left, the coroner ruled against suicide as the cause of death, because they thought that the person who died may have changed their mind after writing the note. We also don't know for certain why some people leave suicide notes and others do not. It may simply be that those who are more communicative in life are more likely to leave a final written message for loved ones.[2]

Given that suicide notes are often not left, how else might we ascertain that a death was self-inflicted? We could consider the person's mental health history, whether they had experienced acute or chronic stressful life events or whether they talked about taking their own life, particularly in the recent past. These are intuitive suggestions, except that interpreting the answers to these questions is challenging. Having a history of mental health problems or experiencing a recent acute stressor are not particularly good markers of suicide risk and the majority of people who talk about suicide will never die by suicide. As we'll see later, although suicide usually happens against the backdrop of mental health problems, the overwhelming majority of people with mental health problems will never die by suicide.[3] Nonetheless, this is what coroners (and their equivalents) around the world do. They try to piece together an individual's life when deciding whether a death is a suicide or not. They gather information about the circumstances surrounding a death and then make a judgement about whether they believe there was sufficient evidence to record a suicide verdict. This is a difficult task.

Legally, personally and culturally, there are also a whole raft of challenges in classifying a death as suicide. The family may not believe that the death was a suicide or wish the death to be classified as such, especially in countries where suicide remains illegal, where it is highly stigmatised or where it has implications for life insurance. The nature of death classification also depends on where the death occurred, as each country has different ascertainment procedures and these are influenced by myriad cultural factors. Even across the four nations of the UK there are marked differences. For example, until 2019, in England and Wales a coroner had to be satisfied 'beyond reasonable doubt' that a person intended to take their own life before recording a death as a suicide. This is the same (high) burden of proof that is required in a criminal court. In addition to the widespread concern that the burden of proof had been too high, leading to the under-reporting of suicides in England and Wales, arguably this crime-like system also added to the stigma around suicide. I was very pleased, therefore, when the High Court in London ruled that suicide verdicts should be treated like civil verdicts, with coroners instructed to make judgements based on 'the balance of probabilities' (lower burden of proof, as in civil law) rather than 'beyond reasonable doubt'.

Fewer than 400 miles north, in Scotland, under Scots law 'the balance of probabilities' has been used by the Crown Office and Procurator Fiscal Service to decide on possible cases of suicide for decades. Incidentally, 25 years ago when I was analysing coroners' inquest papers in Northern Ireland to aid the death registration clerks, I was surprised to learn that one of the coroners would routinely write in pencil on the back of the inquest papers whether he thought a death was a suicide or not. This unofficial note was to aid the clerk in their ascertainment. Aside from the impact on families, the inconsistent classification of death procedures across nations makes it difficult to compare the rates of suicide across different countries. One solution to this has been that in many countries the suicide statistics are reported alongside 'undetermined deaths' or 'deaths by misadventure', as many of the latter are likely to be cases of suicide. The inclusion of probable suicides helps paint a truer picture of the scale of suicides.

Challenges also plague the way in which we define non-fatal self-injurious behaviours such as overdoses and self-cutting.[4] Much of the difficulty lies in being able to accurately ascribe the motives to such behaviours. Most disagreement is around whether a self-injurious act is suicidal, i.e., a suicide attempt, or not, namely non-suicidal injury; or whether it is possible to reliably distinguish between the two kinds of acts. Broadly speaking, different approaches have been adopted in the UK compared to in the USA. So, if someone presents to hospital with medically serious self-cutting in the UK, almost certainly this will appear in their clinical notes as self-harm. Self-harm is the preferred term because it covers all types of intentional self-injury or self-poisoning, irrespective of the motive underlying the behaviour. Indeed the recommended clinical care following any self-injurious behaviour is informed by the National Institute for Health and Care Excellence (NICE) guidelines on the management of self-harm.[5] One of the main reasons why self-harm is used as an umbrella term is because, in part, it overcomes the difficulty in determining whether the self-cutting episode or instance of overdose was suicidal in intent or not. This is important because we know that, when asked, people's motives change over time, they often express multiple motives, and the answers they give can be dependent on who asks the question and whether there are implications for their clinical care.[6] Other times, people are ambivalent or just don't know.

Andrew's story illustrates some of this ambiguity. One evening when he was in his late thirties, Andrew was picked up by a charity after a member of the public alerted them to a man in the local river. The volunteers from the charity managed to rescue him, by which time the emergency services had arrived and were able to transport him to a nearby hospital. After a night's medical observation, he discharged himself from hospital before the liaison psychiatry team had a chance to assess him. When I asked him sometime later why he hadn't waited, I expected him to say because he was fine, that he had had too much to drink the night before and he wouldn't do it again. But he surprised me. He said that he didn't really know why he had done what he did, so why wait? You can see his logic: if he didn't know why, *they* certainly wouldn't know why. Yes, he was mentally exhausted, but he wasn't at rock bottom, like he had been when he had taken an overdose in the past. He was just tired and was 'on a downer' that day, but he didn't think he was suicidal. It was more that he thought he would take his chances and see what happened and if he survived he survived and if he didn't he didn't. He was extremely matter-of-fact. From this brief exchange it is difficult to know whether Andrew's self-harm episode was suicidal in intent or not. Nonetheless, what is clear is that, irrespective of his motives, his actions could have ended his life.

If we look to our colleagues in the USA, they adopt a different stance about what constitutes a suicidal act. They tend not to use the term self-harm, preferring to describe self-injurious behaviours dichotomously as either a suicide attempt (when suicidal intent is present) or as non-suicidal self-injury (when the motive is something other than ending life). And for the reasons outlined above, this has been a bone of contention across the Atlantic. The American approach, however, has the advantage of catering for those people who are adamant that their self-cutting was definitely not motivated by suicidal intent. Indeed, some people are offended when their non-suicidal self-injury is lumped together with suicide attempts. For them, their self-cutting is a means of coping with their pain. Perhaps counter-intuitively, it is a means of staying alive and most definitely not a suicide attempt. But what about those who conceal their suicidal intent or who are unsure or are ambivalent? As this debate is not likely to be resolved any-time soon, for the purposes of this book, when I talk about self-harm, I am referring to any self-injurious behaviours, irrespective of motive. When I mention suicidal behaviour, suicide attempts or non-suicidal self-injury, it means that I am more certain of the motives that did or did not drive the behaviour.

## Who Is At Risk of Suicide?

Suicide is among the top 20 leading causes of death worldwide and is the second leading cause of death among 15–29-year-olds.[7] It accounts for 1.5 per cent of all mortality, globally. In terms of the regions of the world, suicide ranks in the top ten leading causes of death in eastern Europe, central Europe, Australasia, and parts of Asia Pacific and North America.[8] More than three quarters (79 per cent) of the world's suicides are in low- and middle-income countries, with 60 per cent of all suicides being in Asia.[9] Paradoxically, the rates of suicide are lower in low- and middle-income countries relative to high-income countries, but they comprise a larger proportion of the world's suicide deaths as they have a larger population size. Despite the fact that globally the vast majority of suicides occur in low- and middle-income countries, the sad reality is that most of the published research evidence is from high-income countries. All too often the suicide prevention research field has blindly applied Western high-income country understandings of suicide to low- and middle-income contexts. This is clearly inappropriate. If we are to truly tackle suicide as a global public health priority much more needs to be done to redress this imbalance. We must develop more contextually and culturally sensitive programmes of suicide prevention research. In addition, we need to routinely involve people with lived experience of bereavement by suicide as well as those with a history of suicidal thoughts and behaviours in suicide prevention research and its implementation in practice.

In almost every country in the world, more men die by suicide than women and, in Western countries, men are as much as three times more likely to take their own lives than women.[10] For example, in the UK, three quarters of suicides are male and recent statistics from the USA show that the suicide rate for men is 3.7 times that of women.[11] In terms of broad brushes, the male to female ratio tends to be greatest in the countries of Europe and in the Americas, and lowest in Southeast Asia and the western Pacific region. In terms of why male suicide outstrips that of females, there is no one simple explanation. However, the reasons will include use of more lethal methods of suicide, differential rates of help-seeking, cultural norms and expectations around masculinity, the male association with alcohol and the impact on men of loss of intimate relationships.[12]

Regarding suicide rates by country, using the most recent data from the WHO, Guyana, Lithuania, Russia and Kazakhstan report suicide rates that are among the highest globally. By contrast, countries such as Jamaica, Antigua, Syria and the Maldives consistently report the lowest suicide rates.[13] There is also huge variation within continents. Let's take Europe as an example – we have Lithuania (25.7 per 100,000) and Russia (26.5 per 100,000) at the top of the unenviable league table of suicide rates and Greece (3.8 per 100,000) and Italy (5.5 per 100,000) with some of the lowest rates of suicide in Europe. When we are drawing national comparisons, we need to be cautious because each country records suicide deaths differently and there are many cultural, religious and political pressures on whether or not deaths are recorded as suicide. Moreover, even the WHO struggles to obtain up-to-date and reliable data from many countries in the world.

From a global perspective, the rates of suicide are highest among older adults, in particular those aged 70 years and older. Although the rates are higher, suicide is not a leading cause of death in this age group because most people will die from other causes such as cancer, cardiovascular disease and dementia.[14] Conversely, whereas the rates of suicide among young people are numerically lower than those who are middle-aged or older, suicide is one of the leading causes of death in young people. In the USA, suicide is the second leading cause of death among those aged between 10 and 34 years of age.[15] Globally, suicide is also the second leading cause of death in young people aged 15–29 years, after road traffic injury. In the UK, suicide is the leading cause of death for men aged 35–49 years, and the leading cause of death for men and women aged 20–34 years.[16] In recent years, the suicide rates of young people have been on the increase, especially among young females. Part of the explanation for this increase is because more females have switched to more lethal methods of suicide. Contrary to global trends, the latest data from the UK suggest that rates of suicide are highest in those aged 45–49 years, even higher than older adults. Whereas suicide rates have been decreasing in all age groups in China, India's rates have been characterised by a fall in youth suicide but an increase among older adults.[17]

Although I've highlighted some international comparisons, suicide and suicide attempt rates are not static and are affected by social and economic changes. Indeed, the latest data from the UK, USA, Brazil and Australia point to increasing rates of suicide in these countries in recent years whereas there have been notable deceases in the suicide rates in other countries, such as Sri Lanka, Hungary and India. From a global perspective, since 1990, although absolute numbers of people who are dying from suicide have increased (by about 7 per cent over the 27 years studied, up until 2016 – the latest data available), the suicide rate, that is, the proportion of people who die per population, has decreased by about one third. This decrease has been lower in men compared to women and largely accounted for by falls in China and, to less of a degree, decreases in India.[18]

It is difficult to accurately estimate the number of non-fatal suicide attempts. However, the WHO says that for every death by suicide, about 20 people will make a non-fatal suicide attempt.[19] This translates into 16 million suicide attempts globally each year. In many countries, such attempts are most common in those aged 18–34 years. Women tend to attempt suicide more frequently than men.[20] Suicide attempts as well as deaths by suicide are rare before puberty.[21] In a recent study of adolescents from 59 low- and middle-income countries, 16.9 per cent reported suicidal ideation and 17 per cent reported suicide attempts in the previous 12 months.[22] By comparison, in another cross-national study of more than 52,000 people from high-income as well as low- and middle-income countries, overall 2 per cent of people reported suicide ideation in the previous 12 months, whereas 0.5 per cent had attempted suicide in the same time period.[23] But in the World Mental Health Survey, the most comprehensive study to date of suicidal thoughts and behaviours in adults, the lifetime rate of suicide ideation was 9.2 per cent with 2.7 per cent of adults reporting a suicide attempt at some time in their past.[24] In short, despite the international differences in rates, what is clear is that suicide and suicide attempts can affect millions of us as we journey from adolescence through adulthood.

## Health inequalities

Despite not knowing all of the reasons why there are such variations in national and international suicide rates, without question, health inequalities are central to any explanation. Health inequalities are systematic differences in health outcomes between social groups where those from more socially disadvantaged groups live shorter lives and experience more ill health. In essence, the greater the health inequality, the greater the risk of suicide. Health inequality is deeply rooted in societies and over many decades social and healthcare policies have contributed to an exacerbation in these adverse outcomes. These inequalities may also be related to ethnicity, sexuality or gender identity, such that any policy that contributes to stigma, shame, defeat and entrapment may have an adverse impact on one's mental health. For example, although we know that lesbian, gay, bisexual or trans people are at higher suicide risk than heterosexual or cisgender groups, more needs to be done to understand and address these stark inequalities.[25]

When considering issues around inequality, this must include a close examination of the relationship between socioeconomic inequalities and suicide. Socioeconomic inequalities can be measured in many different ways, but indicators such as social class, occupation, educational level, income or whether you own a house or not are often used. Steve Platt, a good friend and health policy researcher from the University of Edinburgh, has dedicated much of his career to understanding the nature of this relationship. In a chapter he wrote for *The International Handbook of Suicide Prevention*, he reviewed the worldwide literature and concluded that there was evidence across a wide range of indicators of an inverse relationship between socioeconomic disadvantage and suicide risk.[26] In addition, using data from Scotland, he illustrated the extent of this inequality. People in the lowest social class who lived in the most deprived areas were about ten times more likely to die by suicide compared to those in the highest social class living in the most affluent areas. For too long, governments have ignored these inequalities. However, if we are serious about preventing suicide, we need to reduce the health inequalities gap between those with and without social advantage. If we are able to do so, we would go some way to addressing much of the recent increase in suicide in countries such as the UK, USA, Brazil and Australia.

The COVID-19 pandemic has also put the issue of mental health inequality firmly on the international research and public health policy map. In spring 2020, I was part of a group of experts, including people with lived experience of mental health, who published a position paper calling for mental health research to be an integral part of the COVID-19 response.[27] At around the same time, David Gunnell from Bristol University convened the International COVID-19 Suicide Prevention Research Collaboration. The aim of this collaboration was to bring together researchers and others involved in suicide prevention, to avoid duplication and to maximise the impact of suicide prevention research activities globally. In the early days of the pandemic, our collective concern was that national government responses to contain the spread of the disease, for example the lockdown measures, together with the economic costs in terms of people's jobs, could create a perfect storm of suicide risk factors.[28]

Even now, we still don't know what the longer-term effects of the COVID-19 pandemic will be on the global suicide rates, and any effect will likely be different across continents, countries, communities and individuals. If we look to the severe acute respiratory syndrome (SARS) outbreak, another coronavirus that spread across parts of Asia in 2003, the suicide rates increased in older adults but not among younger people during that epidemic – and levels of anxiety, depression and post-traumatic stress also increased. However, the scale of the COVID-19 pandemic has been vast compared to that of SARS.[29]

We also know from past economic recessions that suicide deaths can increase during periods of economic crisis. Take the Great Recession that ravaged Europe and North America between 2008 and 2010 and beyond. In many countries globally, there were high levels of unemployment and widespread financial hardship, especially among those who were already vulnerable. A conservative estimate, published a few years after the recession, suggested that there were 10,000 more suicides than would have been expected in the European Union, Canada and the USA since the start of the financial crisis in 2007.[30] It is clear: recessions can kill. Therefore the continued economic fallout of COVID-19 remains a real concern. Add to this the COVID-19 disruptions to mental health services, the impact of school closures, of social isolation, the increase in domestic violence and the adjustment to new ways of working and socialising – these are all potential risks to our mental health.

We also know from data on suicidal thoughts that COVID-19 has affected the mental health of some groups of people more than others.[31] For example, I have been leading the UK COVID-19 Mental Health and Wellbeing study, a UK-wide study tracking the mental health of adults across the UK since spring 2020. In the first paper to be published from this study, we analysed the data for the first six weeks of the lockdown in the UK after the whole population had been instructed to stay at home, protect the National Health Service (NHS) and save lives.[32] In our study, we asked people about their mental health three times across these six weeks. The findings were disconcerting. As the lockdown continued, the proportion of people in our survey who reported suicidal thoughts increased across these initial six weeks, to almost 10 per cent by the third time of asking. These findings were striking because across the same time period, the levels of symptoms of anxiety decreased and the levels of depressive symptoms stayed about the same. To my mind, these increases in suicidal thoughts during lockdown reflected the economic and social uncertainty caused by the pandemic.

The findings from different groups within our sample were even more troubling. Young people, those with pre-existing mental health problems and those from socially disadvantaged backgrounds were even more affected, reporting higher levels of suicidal thoughts than other groups. Whereas older people were bearing the brunt of the physical effects of the virus, young people's futures were being compromised. When talking about the consequences of COVID-19 the author Damian Barr posted the following tweet in April 2020: 'We are not all in the same boat. We are all in the same storm. Some are on super-yachts. Some have just the one oar.' Damian Barr's tweet rings true. We are not all in it together.

The suicidal thoughts data mentioned above relate to the early phase of the pandemic in the UK. It will be several years before we have the full picture of the impact of COVID-19 on suicide and suicidal behaviour. My wider apprehension, though, is that we will be living with the consequences of COVID-19 for a long time to come as the world continues to recover from its effects.[33] Consequently, we need to ensure workforce safety nets are in place to buffer people from the impacts of the pandemic-induced economic storm. We also need to do more to help those who have been most affected, including women, those with pre-existing mental health problems, young people and those who are socially disadvantaged. I am confident, though, that if we continue to act together nationally and internationally we will be able to mitigate the longer-term impact of COVID-19.

## Words Matter

People use many different phrases to describe people who self-harm, attempt suicide or die by suicide. However, we need to be careful because the language we use may cause distress or offence and add to the stigma experienced by family members of those who have died by suicide as well as by those who have attempted suicide. Let's consider the phrase 'committed suicide'. It is widely used, being part and parcel of our national discourse on suicide in pubs, in clubs, on the news, online, in films and on the TV. We hear it everywhere. However, for some, this phrase is offensive and its use is insensitive and distressing because it harks back to a time when suicide was considered a criminal act. And this was not that long ago in some countries. In the UK, the Suicide Act, decriminalising suicide, was passed in 1961 and it wasn't until 1993 that the Criminal Law (Suicide) Act was passed, doing the same, in Ireland. Even more concerning, though, is that suicide remains a criminal offence in many countries across the globe including Bangladesh, Malaysia and Saudi Arabia. Reflecting the growing discourse and awareness, there are international media reporting guidelines that are explicit in recommending against the use of the term, which I'll return to later in the book (see page 32). But the debate has moved beyond the traditional media reporting: indeed, taking a recent example from popular culture, there have been numerous calls for Lin-Manuel Miranda to change the lyrics of the song 'Alexander Hamilton' from the hit Broadway musical *Hamilton,* which features the line 'the cousin committed suicide', to 'the cousin died by suicide'. Others argue that the debate around the use of the verb 'commit', despite being well-intentioned, is simplistic and does not take sufficient account of context.[34]

Turning to self-harm and suicide attempts, pejorative language, like 'it's only attention-seeking and manipulative', is still used too often. It needs to be eliminated and I discuss wider issues related to 'attention-seeking' in Chapter 3 (page 56). To my mind, it is simple. Imagine the mental pain that someone must be experiencing if they'll inflict physical pain on themselves, often in an effort to gain relief. Is that attention-seeking? Of course it is not, it is attention-needing and it is definitely not done to *simply* seek attention. However, if you are asking whether a person is trying to draw attention to their distress, well then, the answer is yes, they are. They are trying to draw attention to the pain they are experiencing or they don't know how else to express how they are feeling. And our response should be how can we respond with compassion and support rather than with scorn and indignation? Similarly, using the word 'manipulative' is unacceptable. It misses the complexity of the motives that drive any behaviour and crucially it also misses the point that every one of us manipulates the people around us every single day.[35] Any utterance or action that we undertake which seeks to achieve a particular end is manipulative. So never mind the offence caused, it just does not make any sense to label people who self-harm as such.

The language issue is complex though, as illustrated by a recent online study led by Prianka Padmanathan from the University of Bristol and colleagues at Samaritans and the University of Nottingham.[36] They asked people, including those who had been directly affected by suicide, about their attitudes to different descriptions of suicidal behaviour and to rate how acceptable they thought each description was. The findings were interesting, but some were also quite surprising. First, but not unexpected, the majority of people rated the terms 'ended their life', 'died by suicide' and 'took their own life' as being most 'acceptable'. When asked, some people said that they rated these more positively because they reflect the fact that the person 'chose to do it' [take their own life], thereby acknowledging that the person who died had agency, that they had made a decision to end their life. But they also thought that such descriptions weren't 'too harsh' and that, in the words of one person, it 'keeps her human'. Conversely, phrases such as 'topped themselves', 'successful suicide', and 'completed suicide' were much more likely to be rated as unacceptable and are therefore best avoided. For example, the majority of people who commented disliked 'successful suicide' as it framed suicide positively and was insensitive and could cause distress.

Of particular interest and quite surprising was the fact that people were split in terms of their rating of 'committed suicide'. Some rated it as most acceptable and others thought it was not acceptable at all. For those who rated it as acceptable, some did so because they thought it was an accurate description of the act or because it was commonly used. Others didn't agree that the term implied criminality. Of all the terms that people rated, 'committed suicide' attracted the biggest differences in acceptability scores. People clearly have strong feelings about using this phrase. One parent who had lost their son to suicide expressed anger at the perceived chastisement by suicide researchers for using this term. Their view contrasts with those of others who have campaigned against the use of this term (full disclosure: I have been vocal against using the term 'committed suicide' for several years). The parent felt that it was political correctness gone too far and that no one has the right to correct them when they are describing their son's death. Of course, their view is completely valid and highlights that the issue around language isn't straightforward and loved ones are entitled to use whatever language they are comfortable with. However, given the potential for some people to become distressed, I personally avoid using the term 'committed suicide' entirely now. Indeed, I regularly meet bereaved parents, partners and other family members who find the use of the term disrespectful, distressing and stigmatising. A woman whose husband took his own life recently told me that she is taken aback and actually has a physiological response when she hears the phrase 'committing suicide' on the news or hears someone around her say it. She has to catch her breath, though she admitted: 'I don't really know why, it just sounds really harsh and cold.' As a result, this is the only section in this book where the phrase appears. Needless to say, irrespective of your standpoint, this issue should be dealt with sensitively and compassionately.

# What Suicidal Pain Feels Like

BEFORE MOVING ON to the risk factors for suicide and suicide attempts, it is useful to get some sense of what suicidal pain feels like. Over the course of my career, bereaved relatives have sent me their loved ones' final letters, notes or diaries, often written in the moments before death. This is a huge honour, but it is also an immense responsibility. Family members hope that these personal communications will provide a window into their son's, daughter's or partner's thinking in the final moments before they took their own life. In some cases they do, they are very clear, detailed and explicit; in other cases, they are not, simply outlining a set of will-like instructions. Also, when examined in isolation, it can be difficult to distil the complex motivations underpinning any suicide. However, most often the notes are powerful documents, conveying the pain of suicide and the sense of failure that often precedes the decision to end one's life.[1] Here is a note I received a few years ago, written by Jamie, a middle-aged man. It communicates his sense of failure and his black-and-white thinking, both of which often characterise the suicidal state:

If you are reading this, I have had enough and I'm dead. You can see how bollocks my life is. I can't think of any day when things have gone well recently and who really cares about me anyway. I am a failure, can do nothing right. Useless. Trapped. With [name of girlfriend], I was really happy, for once in my life!! I tried my hardest with her and I was shit and I still failed. What did she want, I didn't know what to do?

It is difficult not to identify with Jamie. We have all experienced the pain of a relationship breakdown, we have all felt useless and a failure at some time or another. Clearly, we know nothing about Jamie's past, his background, his mental health or what else was going on in his life. Looking beyond his suicide note, therefore, the challenge is to understand how and why the pain he was experiencing became so much that he felt that his life was not worth living. One clue may be in his use of the word 'trapped'. As I will discuss throughout this book, I believe that being trapped by unbearable pain is key to understanding suicide as I consider it to be central to the final common pathway to suicide.

The focus on Jamie's failed relationship also highlights what I sometimes describe as the 'everydayness' of suicide. I don't mean to downplay the drivers of suicide. By this I mean that what leads someone to become suicidal is very often about what happens every day: everyday failures, everyday crises and everyday losses. Too often people think that suicide is about the out-of-the-ordinary, a response to things that happen to other people and not to them, when it is not. For some, suicide is about bullying, divorce, the loss of a job. For others, it is about bereavement, bankruptcy, shame, discrimination, loss of benefits or illness. It is about how we respond to stressful events and circumstances as well as the cards that we are dealt at birth. But it is important to remember that suicide is never inevitable. It is preventable right up until the final moment.

Still too often when I am talking to someone about suicide, especially to someone who has no direct experience of it, it becomes apparent that they believe people who kill themselves are different from them. It is as if they believe that there is a particular type of person who kills themselves, and that they are not that type of person – they believe that they are, in some way, inoculated against suicide. They are not. Of course I understand this 'othering', this distancing from suicide; it helps them to feel protected, perhaps. But the fact is that this is simply untrue and serves only to fuel the stigma, and it needs to be challenged. Suicide can affect any one of us; there is no vaccine against suicide. There are some groups of people who are more at risk of suicide than others, but suicide affects women as well as men, young people as well as older people, Black people, white people, married people and single people.[2]

Ever since my earliest days working on suicide, I've been interested in suicide notes because, despite their constraints, they provide unique insights into acute suicidal pain. When I was in my early twenties with no direct experience of suicide, starting out on my PhD, they really helped me to appreciate what it feels like to be suicidal and not able to see alternatives. They are intensely personal documents. One of the first suicide notes that I ever read was from a 16-year-old boy who took his own life close to where he lived. His act was seemingly impulsive. He'd been drinking and he'd had an argument with his mother because his school had called her earlier that day, saying that he'd been in a fight with someone in his class. This wasn't the first time. She confronted him and this led to a really heated argument, and he stormed out of the house. When he didn't return later that night, she went out searching for him; but her efforts were in vain as, tragically, a few hours later, the police found him, dead.

It felt like I knew him, as I had learned about his short life, his traumatic childhood and his struggle with drugs and alcohol, from reading the coroner's inquest files. I spent all of that summer in Belfast examining inquest papers of potential deaths by suicide, in an effort to identify patterns in the suicides. His file was among the first batch of potential suicides that I reviewed. When I came across it, I remember thinking he was about the same age as my youngest brother and a wave of sadness came over me as I thought how unfair life was. Unlike my brother, he had been through hell. I was sitting at my desk in the imposing Court House in Belfast, where the coroner's office was, leafing through statements from his mother, his GP and his social worker. I remember it well – I was coming towards the end of the documents in his file and I was taken aback as I came across his photograph and his suicide note bound together with a paper clip. There was something about the paper clip that struck me as so sad. It was so impersonal. His note was brief, but stark. In shaky handwriting, it simply said that he knew she – his mother – would always be angry with him. This tunnel vision, not being able to see a time when things will be different, is very common in suicide notes and suicidal communications more generally. That was it. His whole existence reduced to one sentence. When I got home that night I wept.

That note was part of a wider study of suicide notes that I conducted for my PhD.[3] It was a relatively small study, where I developed psychological profiles of suicidal individuals by analysing suicide notes that I had uncovered in the inquest papers. This involved coding what people had written into different themes. The hope was that if we had more fine-grained profiles we could better identify those at risk of suicide. Although the analyses are well over 20 years old, the key findings are still as relevant today to understanding suicide as they were then. In over 90 per cent of the notes, the person who died talked about their unbearable psychological pain and their desire for an urgent and permanent solution. One of the notes, written by Dave, conveys this intensity and urgency:

> I just cannot go on, I've had enough.
> Life is too much, you are better off without me
> My head is going to explode. I need it to end.
> I've had too much pain. I am just so sorry. I cannot do it.
> I love you, this has nothing to do with you.

Dave was in his early twenties when he died. Like the vast majority of people who die by suicide, he had not been in touch with mental health services in the year before his death.[4] In fact, he had never been in contact with mental health services. Although he had been drinking before he died, he hadn't drunk that much. He had only ever had one long-term girlfriend, but the relationship had been strained in the preceding months. He had also recently lost his grandmother, to whom he was close, who had died from a stroke. In the weeks before his death, his parents had put his low mood down to the bereavement and also to the fact that he had been anxious about forthcoming university exams. Although he had told them that he wasn't sleeping very well, they were unaware of any relationship issues.

What is important to recognise about Dave's final words is that he doesn't talk about wanting to end his life. As I mentioned earlier, suicide is not usually about the desire to die, it's about ending the unbearable mental pain. Dave was mentally exhausted. It is likely that the stress of losing his grandmother, his relationship concerns and his exam worries were made even worse by his difficulties sleeping. Good-quality sleep is vital to a healthy existence.[5] Poor sleep makes it much more challenging to think clearly, to deal with life's obstacles, to see options, to keep things in perspective and to manage your mood.

We should never overlook the importance of sleep to our well-being. As Dave's story highlights, sleep disturbance is a recognised risk factor for suicidal thoughts and behaviours. For example, in a study led by Mari Hysing and Borge Sivertsen of 10,000 adolescents in Norway, we found a clear relationship between sleep and self-harm.[6] We found a dose-response relationship; the more

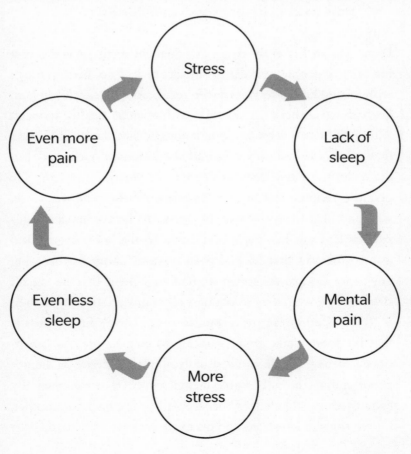

sleep problems, the higher frequency of self-harm. Numerous academic reviews of the relationship between sleep disturbances and the full range of suicidal behaviours have been published in recent years.[7] They all come to the same conclusion: that sleep disturbance is associated with suicide and self-harm risk. They also suggest that sleep disturbance may increase suicide risk as it contributes to psychiatric disorder and impulsivity, as well as affecting decision-making and emotion regulation.

It is so easy to fall into a damaging, vicious cycle of negative thoughts that are driven by stress and mental pain.

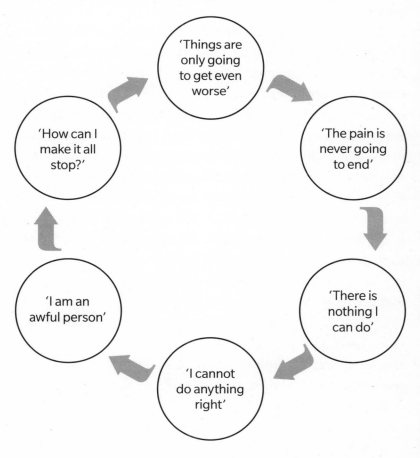

For some, these cycles escalate and escalate until suicide seems to be an option, the only option, the ultimate solution to stopping the debilitating thoughts. One of the founders of modern suicide research, Edwin Shneidman, talked about suicide as a permanent solution to often temporary problems.[8] He was so right, and Dave's story seems to typify this description. Dave clearly articulates the overwhelming nature of his pain when he says: 'My head is going to explode. I need it to end. I've had too much pain.' So if we try to make sense of what drives someone to suicide, we should think about their pain – pain that, for many, may be hidden.

People attempt suicide or take their own lives when they can see no end to their pain, when they feel trapped by it and that there is no way out.[9] Like physical pain, there is only so much mental pain that we can withstand and, when we reach our limit, something has to give. Sadly, for too many people, it is life that gives. Dave's comment 'you are better off without me' is also really telling. Many people who are suicidal think they are a burden to others and that if they kill themselves then their loved ones will be better off. So rather than seeing suicide as a selfish act, paradoxically, in the mind of the person who is consumed by pain, it is quite the opposite. They feel that they are doing their loved ones a favour.

After a recent talk I gave in London, a mother who had lost her daughter, Jen, sent me her suicide note, in the hope that it could help with my research. Jen was 34 when she died. Once again, it is difficult to read. Like Dave's and Jamie's letters, in an excerpt from her note, Jen conveys her pain, but this time her mental pain is compounded by physical pain. She writes:

. . . I have just had enough of all of this pain, I cannot go on anymore. The only pleasure that I have gotten out of living recently is walking Benny [the dog], and now I am in so much physical pain that I just cannot even do that. There is just nothing that I can do. I just need to be free from all of this pain and I just cannot think of any other way out. My life is just so meaningless and empty.

The overwhelming nature of her pain is obvious when Jen says 'I have just had enough of all of this pain' and later adds that 'I just need to be free from all of this pain'. Her experience fits with the findings of one of our research studies led by Katerina Kavalidou where we found physical as well as mental pain to be associated with suicidal ideation.[10] Jen's feeling of complete powerlessness is also apparent when she says that there is nothing she can do about the pain. Similarly, she also communicates her inability to see a future without pain. Her tunnel vision and perceiving suicide as 'I just cannot think of any other way out' are akin to 'calling cards' of the suicidal mind. The common theme permeating all three of the notes is entrapment; Jamie, Dave and Jen were all trapped by pain, and their deaths were driven by the all-consuming wish to escape it. Hopefully you'll see a recurrent theme emerging: suicide and entrapment are inextricably linked. I'll talk more about entrapment in Chapter 6 (page 89).

I was also really struck by Jen's final line. To me, it is a rallying call for all of us. We all have a duty, a responsibility, as a society to do whatever we can so that people around us don't feel such emptiness and meaninglessness, don't feel so disconnected, that they see suicide as the only way to be free.

## The Importance of Social Connection

Anthropologists and sociologists have characterised suicide statistics historically as an index of the 'sickness' of a society.[11] Although I wouldn't use the term sickness, I think these social scientists are on to something with that description. Suicides are an awful indictment on society. It is unacceptable that we live in a world where so many people, like Jamie, Dave and Jen, see no other option but to end their lives. And too often their deaths are hastened because they don't think that they are valued or valuable. I am writing this section on World Suicide Prevention Day (WSPD) in 2020, which is the culmination of global efforts to raise awareness around suicide and suicide prevention annually. Organised under the auspices of the International Association for Suicide Prevention (IASP), WSPD happens on 10 September every year and it serves as a regular reminder of the scale of the challenge that we face. Despite my being a strong advocate of WSPD, we must remember that it is only one day in the year, and clearly suicide prevention efforts need to be 24/7, 365 days each and every year.

Returning to the idea of being valued and valuable, the theme of WSPD in 2020 was 'working together to prevent suicide' and, as part of the day's activities, the IASP produced a short film entitled *Step Closer*.[12] The imagery was evocative and spoke to the importance of human connection. Its message was simple: it encouraged all of us to take a step closer, to make connections, knowing that by connecting or reconnecting with another human being we could help to save a life.

The opening clip of the video reminds us that we can all play a part in preventing suicide. It illustrated this through the

# 3

# Myths and Misunderstandings

TWENTY YEARS AGO, not only was suicide rarely talked about in the media beyond sensationalised headlines, but it was also infrequently discussed openly in families, communities or workplaces. When it was considered, it was talked about in hushed tones. Arguably, this absence of significant public or private discourse has contributed to the stigma and the reinforcement of the many myths around suicide. Indeed, in my view, these myths, such as 'asking someone about suicide will plant the idea into their head', have continued to be propagated unchecked and only fairly recently have they been challenged in a meaningful way in the mainstream media and elsewhere.

We have made considerable strides forward in terms of challenging these myths in the last few years, but I am continually surprised by how persistent they are. By way of illustration, I gave my first public talk on suicide in Belfast, Northern Ireland, in the late nineties. At that talk, I listed 14 commonly reported myths that I had gleaned from classic texts on suicide. In the Q&A session after the talk, we discussed each myth in turn, examining who held which myth and why. And it quickly became apparent that most members of the audience admitted to believing most of the myths. When I asked them where they had come across these myths, it tended to be hearsay; talking to their friends or family, from something that they had seen on TV or read in a newspaper or a magazine (no one mentioned the Internet, as it was only in its infancy then).

Now, fast forward to 2019. I was doing a couple of talks in England, similar to the one I did in Belfast all those years before, and once again the audiences comprised members of the general public. After several years of not discussing myths in my presentations, I had reintroduced my 'suicide myths' slide to see whether we had made any progress in dispelling them. I had made no substantial changes to the text and used the same format as before: we chatted through the myths, one by one, with me probing which of the myths the audience thought were true and why. And although it is a little unfair to make a direct comparison, from the discussion it was clear that, although the public discourse around suicide has improved beyond recognition since the nineties, the vast majority of myths still persisted and we have a long way to go in terms of smashing the generations-old beliefs around suicide.

I have listed the myths below in no particular order. Why not go through each of the myths and ask yourself whether you think they are true? I guarantee that there will be at least some that you think are statements of fact. I'll then take you through each myth in turn and explain why they are myths and how some are less clear-cut than others.

### Those who talk about suicide are not at risk of suicide

This first myth is embedded in the idea that if someone is intent on ending their life then the last thing they will do is tell anyone that they are thinking of suicide. This is false and misses the

## MYTHS ABOUT SUICIDE

1. Those who talk about suicide are not at risk of suicide.
2. All suicidal people are depressed or mentally ill.
3. Suicide occurs without warning.
4. Asking about suicide 'plants' the idea in someone's head.
5. Suicidal people clearly want to die.
6. When someone becomes suicidal they will always remain suicidal.
7. Suicide is inherited.
8. Suicidal behaviour is motivated by attention-seeking.
9. Suicide is caused by a single factor.
10. Suicide cannot be prevented.
11. Only people of a particular social class die by suicide.
12. Improvement in emotional state means lessened suicide risk.
13. Thinking about suicide is rare.
14. People who attempt suicide by a low-lethality means are not serious about killing themselves.

complexity of the motives that underpin suicide, not to mention the ambivalence and the waxing and waning nature of suicidal thoughts and urges.[1] By talking about suicide they may also be reaching out for help. Sadly, I have lost track of the number of times that people have asked me about this, certain that this myth is true.

Over the years, I have been told too many heartbreaking stories where a mother, a father, a partner or a friend has taken comfort from the 'fact' that their loved one was safe because they had talked openly about their suicidal urges. They had been falsely reassured by the myth. Devastatingly, though, in too many instances, their loved ones did go on to take their own lives.

This myth is pervasive, as I have heard similar accounts from GPs and mental health professionals, who have also held such views and who have lost patients or clients to suicide. The estimates vary; however, the reality is that at least four in ten people who die by suicide have talked to someone about taking their own life in advance of doing so.[2] Sometimes such conversations are fleeting; other times, they are more in-depth. Sometimes they are about being tired of living; other times they are more direct, the loved one being explicit in their desire to end their life. The advice is simple. Irrespective of the nature of the communication, take every suicidal utterance seriously. Ask directly and compassionately, then explore what is driving the thoughts of suicide and work together with the person to help to keep them safe. If you don't think you can keep someone safe, always contact a healthcare professional or the emergency services. I provide some practical guidance on asking about suicide and keeping someone safe in Parts 3 and 4.

## All suicidal people are depressed or mentally ill

Although it is often stated in the research literature that 90 per cent of those who die by suicide are depressed or mentally ill, there is growing recognition that this statistic may be an overestimate.[3] Indeed, some have even questioned the legitimacy of this as a so-called established truth in suicide research.[4] Nonetheless, despite the disagreement on the extent of the relationship, most people do agree that suicide usually occurs in the context of mental illness. The mental illnesses most commonly associated with suicide are major depressive disorder, schizophrenia, bipolar disorder and substance use disorders.[5] However, mental illness is neither a prerequisite nor a sufficient cause for suicide and we need to look beyond it to fully understand suicide. Even where mental illness is part of the perfect storm of suicide risk factors, on its own it does not explain why a particular individual dies by suicide.[6] What is more, if we look internationally – for example, to Asia – the association between suicide and mental illness is much weaker than that reported in Western countries. It is estimated that only 35–40 per cent of those who died by suicide in India and China had been diagnosed with depression before death.[7] Therefore, given that more than 60 per cent of the world's suicides occur in Asia and 79 per cent in low- or middle-income countries, it is clearly incorrect to say that all suicidal people are depressed or mentally ill.[8] And even in Western countries, it is not true to say that all people who die by suicide have a mental illness, although many will have. It is also worth noting that suicide frequently happens in the context of social disadvantage and it is often preceded by a sudden loss or the experience of a stressful life event, or it may be an impulsive act; and in these cases there may be no evidence of mental illness.

## Suicide occurs without warning

I find this third myth tricky because, although there are warning signs for suicide (e.g., getting one's affairs in order), they are often difficult to spot in the heat of our everyday lives and, of course, warning signs appear blindingly obvious with hindsight, when we have already lost a loved one. Add into the mix that there are many people who are getting their affairs in order but are not thinking about suicide at all. Also, for a minority of people, there do not appear to be any warning signs. It is even more difficult to identify warning signs if you are caring for someone who lives with suicidal thoughts on a daily basis. In such cases, it is not so much about identifying who is at risk; rather it is about pinpointing when a loved one is especially vulnerable. We are trying to identify what Edwin Shneidman has described as 'death day' – the day when someone would take their own life.[9] However, the sad reality is that we are no better than chance at predicting suicide, warnings or not.[10] Nonetheless, this still remains in the myths section because, although difficult to spot, there are warning signs for suicide (see page 202).

## Asking about suicide 'plants' the idea in someone's head

This myth is the one I have been asked about most often in my career. So, let's be crystal clear: there is *no* evidence that asking someone whether they are suicidal plants the idea in their head. What is more, it may even have the opposite *protective* effect. A few years ago, researchers from King's College London reviewed all of the studies that had examined whether asking about suicide induces suicidal thinking in adults and adolescents and in general as well as in clinical populations.[11] Their findings were unequivocal: asking about suicide does not increase suicidal thinking and in fact it may be associated with reduced suicidal thinking and improvements in mental health. In short, if you are concerned about someone, please ask them directly whether they have been thinking about suicide. It could help them to get the help that they need and, potentially, it could save their life. Talking about suicide may also give people the opportunity to consider their options and rethink their decision to end their life. Of course, as noted above, asking this question is difficult and scary, so I have provided tips on doing so, based on best practice, in Chapter 12.

### Suicidal people clearly want to die

No, they do not. Debunking this myth was one of the first things I learned about the suicidal mind when I embarked on my research career. As a first-year PhD student, I devoured everything I could find that had been written by Edwin Shneidman. He was one of the founders of the American Association of Suicidology, as well as being a pioneer in understanding the suicidal mind. In his seminal book, *Definition of Suicide* (published in 1985), I remember coming across his 'ten commonalities of suicide' for the first time and learning about the myths around suicide.[12] Shneidman's sixth commonality, or common feature, of suicide is especially relevant here as it states that 'the common cognitive state in suicide is ambivalence'. In other words, ambivalence is a key way in which people who are suicidal think. And this is so true; people who are suicidal often cycle between wanting to live and wanting to die. For some, this cycling is almost instantaneous, flipping between wanting to live, then wanting to die and then back to wanting to live again within minutes. For others, this cycling can take hours or days.

People who have survived a suicide attempt often report this ambivalence or desire to live as well as a desire to die and, for some, the life instinct kicks in as soon as they have embarked on a suicide attempt. Kevin Hines, one of the few people to survive jumping from the Golden Gate Bridge in San Francisco, often talks about his immediate regret as soon as he jumped.[13] When he describes his suicide attempt, he recounts vividly how the millisecond after his hands left the railing, he had the instant recognition that he had made the biggest mistake of his life. Despite suffering horrendous injuries, he survived and is now one of the leading mental health campaigners in the US.

For others, like Amir, a man in his sixties whom I met a few years ago and who has survived multiple suicide attempts, it is different. He finds it difficult to disentangle wanting to live and wanting to die because he often experiences both thoughts at the same time. He also thinks that, for him, his suicide attempts are more to do with exhaustion or being overwhelmed. He just wants the 'noises in his head' to stop and he thinks the never-ending thoughts of worthlessness feed his ambivalence about living. Also, his experiences of being suicidal and ambivalent have been different for each of his previous attempts.

On the first occasion, when he was in his mid-twenties, he had been drinking heavily on the night of the suicide attempt and his ambivalence was linked to the termination of a long-term relationship – 'the love of his life' – that had ended abruptly. He was devastated when his girlfriend left him and he couldn't see beyond the emotional pain that he was experiencing. His ambivalence was driven by the belief that he would never find love again, so, to his mind, he may as well die because life was not worth living unless he had someone to share it with. He remembers waking up in hospital the morning after his attempt, groggy but adamant that he hadn't wanted to die and that it was an accidental overdose. But he admits now that that was a lie, and that he had wanted to die in the moment, at the time. As he has got older, when he has been suicidal, the overriding thoughts have been less to do with living or dying and more to do with making the pain stop. He's still ambivalent, though now his ambivalence is directed at himself and he is fixated on whether he deserves to live or not. Of course, for those who have ended their life, we can never know for certain whether they were no longer ambivalent, so exhausted with life that they just really wanted to die.

## When someone becomes suicidal they will always remain suicidal

For most people, suicide risk is usually short-term and linked to a specific situation, often an interpersonal crisis. While suicidal thoughts may come back again for some people, the vast majority will make a full recovery, they will never attempt suicide and will not die by suicide. This reminds me of Dale, in his mid-fifties, who took part in one of our clinical studies after attempting suicide multiple times over a three-month period. He and his family were understandably concerned things would never change and that he'd remain suicidal for the long term. Thankfully, when we were in touch with him again for one of our follow-up sessions, he was doing well. He had started taking medication for his depressive symptoms and was also seeing a psychologist who was helping him to work through his struggles around self-esteem and feelings of worthlessness. As he said to us: 'When I think back to the depths of despair I felt all those months ago, at that time, I just couldn't see a way out, or any end to my suicidal thoughts.' Whereas now he is sleeping so much better and feels in control of his life, and he hasn't felt suicidal for several months.

This is such a powerful message to hold on to if a loved one is in the midst of a suicidal crisis and you fear that things will never improve. They can and they do. But it is important to reach out so that your loved one gets the help that they need.

## Suicide is inherited

Once again, this is one of the more ambiguous myths. On one level it is clearly a myth because the act of taking one's life is, first and foremost, a behaviour and one cannot inherit a behaviour. Nonetheless, as one's vulnerability to suicide is, in part, genetic, then suicide *risk* is, in part, inherited. Indeed, some estimates from twin and adoption studies suggest that suicide has a heritability quotient of 30–50 per cent, although it is somewhat lower when psychiatric illness is accounted for.[14] The heritability quotient is the percentage of variability in a specific characteristic (in this case suicide) that can be explained by genetic factors. I think that when describing the relationship between suicide and heritability, it is more accurate to say that part of the vulnerability to suicide is inherited rather than suicide itself.

## Suicidal behaviour is motivated by attention-seeking

Despite the progress that has been made in destigmatising suicide in recent years, I continue to be dismayed when I hear people talking about this myth. Too often suicidal behaviour and self-harm are described in pejorative terms, with attention-seeking usually being prefixed by 'only' and 'just': for example, 'She [and it is more common that females are stigmatised in this way] has cut herself again, she's just attention-seeking; if she's serious about killing herself, then she'd just do it.' Of course, the suicidal individual is trying to draw attention to their distress, perhaps viewing self-injurious behaviour as the only way to manage it. But this is not 'attention-seeking' in the way that those who are being dismissive suggest. It is a marker of distress, not usually a marker of attention-seeking. For me, it is very simple. Imagine the pain or distress that an individual must be experiencing such that they would inflict pain on themselves as a means of managing or relieving how they are feeling. Every act of self-harm, irrespective of motive, needs to be taken seriously and deserves a compassionate, human response.

About ten years ago, long-standing collaborators and friends, Susan Rasmussen and Keith Hawton, and I conducted the Lifestyle and Wellbeing Study, a large survey of adolescents across Scotland and Northern Ireland.[15] We asked more than 5,500 15–16-year-olds confidentially whether they had self-harmed in the past and, if they had, why they had done so. The findings were concerning, as at least 10 per cent of the young people told us that they had self-harmed at least once in the past, most commonly in the past 12 months. This finding is consistent with other studies internationally.[16] When we enquired about their motives, their responses were eloquent and wide-ranging, and illustrated the complex motivations that underpin self-harm. Below are four that have stuck in my mind and which are relevant because they highlight that self-harm, irrespective of motive, is a manifestation of distress and deserves help and support rather than scorn and dismissal. The first two quotes are from two fifteen-year-olds and they convey that self-harm, for many, is a means of managing one's emotions:

- 'To relieve me of my suffering and pain.'
- 'To take the pain from my heart to my arm.'

The next two quotes are also extremely powerful:

- 'The physical pain rules out the emotional pain.'
- 'Couldn't escape. I just didn't want to live anymore.'

I was really moved the first time I read these latter quotes; I just couldn't shake the thought that these teenagers could see no other alternative to managing their emotional pain. It is heartbreaking to think that these young people had to resort to harming themselves to assuage their pain. Their words are incredibly poignant and I think they highlight that our health comprises both physical and mental health and that they are inextricably linked. There is no mind without body and no body without mind.

### Suicide is caused by a single factor

Without question, suicide is *not* caused by a single factor. Rather, suicide results from a perfect storm of factors and, as I have said already, these factors can be biological, psychological, clinical, social or cultural, and many of them may be hidden.[17] It may seem, when looking from the outside in, that suicide is caused by a single event or factor, but this usually isn't the case. Take, for example, the tragic suicide of the British TV presenter Caroline Flack in February 2020, which attracted extensive media coverage in the UK and beyond. If you listened to much of the mainstream media you would believe that its treatment of Caroline was the sole cause of her untimely death at 40. Or if the media were not being blamed it was the Crown Prosecution Service that was under attack. The reality is that none of us will know for certain what was going through her mind in the hours or minutes before her death, but what is certain is that her untimely death was a personal tragedy likely caused by a multitude of factors unknown to outside observers. Reducing suicide to a single cause helps no one, least of all those who are most at risk of suicide or those left behind following a tragic loss.

## Suicide cannot be prevented

This is a complicated one. At a national level, suicide can be prevented, but it is very difficult to do so.[18] To illustrate, if we inspect the long-term trends in suicide rates across countries and across time, the world's suicide rates have been declining. In statistical terms, we tend to report age-standardised mortality rates and in one recent study Mohsen Naghavi from the University of Washington reported that the age-standardised suicide rates decreased by a third worldwide between 1990 and 2016.[19] This is great news! Indeed, Scotland is a good example of a country that, until recently, had a declining suicide rate. For the ten years up until 2018, the suicide rates decreased year-on-year, culminating in a 20 per cent reduction.[20] So at a country level, this suggests that suicide is preventable. The difficulty, however, is that it isn't clear what accounts for this reduction and it is notoriously difficult to prevent suicide at an individual level.

We do not know for certain whether, or the extent to which, national suicide prevention strategies work or not, but we believe in Scotland's case that the implementation of a ten-year national suicide prevention action plan played some part. However, in other countries, like the USA and Australia, the suicide rates have been increasing in recent years; and in Scotland, after many years of decreases, there has been an increase in the suicide rate since 2018. Irrespective of the explanations for the reductions (or otherwise) at national levels, the ability to prevent suicide on an individual level is even more challenging. As I've said already, we are no better than chance at predicting who will die by suicide.[21] Despite advances in understanding risk and protective factors, the challenge for preventing suicide at the individual level remains; not only are we trying to identify *who* is most likely to take their own lives, but we also need to know *where* and *when* they will do so.

## Only people of a particular social class die by suicide

Suicide is not a respecter of social class. Anyone, irrespective of social class, could die by suicide. The reason why this myth has emerged is because the rates of suicide are higher among those from more disadvantaged backgrounds compared to those who are more affluent. We often talk about the socioeconomic gradient of inequality and, in the case of suicide, this gradient is steep. In the UK, suicide is three times more likely among those who are from the lowest social class compared to those at the top of the social class tree. As I said earlier, suicide is a heartbreaking example of inequality and inequity, and illustrates the importance of taking a public health approach to suicide prevention.[22]

## Improvement in emotional state means lessened suicide risk

This next myth is tinged with sadness because I have met too many people who have lost a loved one to suicide but who had felt falsely reassured because their loved one's emotional state had improved in the days before their death. They harbour guilt because they believe that they had 'let their guard down', that they had failed their loved one because they were not vigilant leading up to the death. Of course, I can understand why a family member or a close friend may feel this way, but it is vital to remember that even with the benefit of hindsight it may not have been possible to save the life of their loved one.

Do not listen to anyone who says that an *improvement in emotional state means lessened suicide risk*. Not only is this a myth, but it may be tragically incorrect, with the inverse relationship being true. It seems that improvement in emotional state is associated with *increased* rather than decreased suicide risk. The logic is as follows: when someone is in the midst of a depressive episode (for example) and overwhelmed with pain, they often do not have the energy or motivation to formulate and enact a suicide plan. However, if they settle upon suicide as the means of ending their pain, then their emotional state may lift as they believe they have *found* the solution to their problems – suicide being the permanent means of ending their pain. The knock-on effect is that, as their emotional state improves, their motivation and energy return and they now have the emotional and cognitive capacity to plan and carry out their suicidal act. If, however, there is a reasonable explanation for the upward shift in mood, that's a relief and there is less of a reason to be vigilant. For example, an individual's mood may improve because they have resolved their crisis, or their medication or psychological treatment is helping them. In such cases, the improvement in emotional state is understandable and welcome, but it is still no guarantee that the person is safe.

The general advice is that if a vulnerable person's mood improves inexplicably, then there is perhaps cause for concern and further probing or support is recommended. Conversations with clinicians over the years have also confirmed the importance of ignoring this myth, with psychiatrists and psychologists reporting tragically that some patients appeared to be much more engaged with treatment and much more content in the days and weeks before they died.

## Thinking about suicide is rare

Sadly, this is not true. Depending on the research study and the population, the prevalence of suicidal thoughts varies extensively. In the World Mental Health Survey, between 3 and 16 per cent of adults internationally report having experienced suicidal thoughts at some stage in their lives.[23] By this I don't mean passive thoughts of suicide such as, 'I am so exhausted I'd like to sleep and not wake up again'; rather I am talking about active thoughts of ending one's life. For example, when we assessed suicidal thinking in over 3,500 young adults (18–34 years old) as part of another study called the Scottish Wellbeing Study, we asked, 'Have you ever seriously thought of taking your life, but not actually attempted to do so?'. The responses highlighted the scale of distress: more than 20 per cent reported having suicidal thoughts at some stage in their lives, with 10 per cent thinking of suicide in the past 12 months.[24] In case you were wondering, the rate of suicidal thoughts is higher if you just focus on young people, as older adults tend to report lower suicidal thoughts.

## People who attempt suicide by a low-lethality means are not serious about killing themselves

This myth relates, in part, to the attention-seeking myth. The idea being that if someone was really serious about ending their own life then they would 'do it right' and choose a really lethal method rather than a so-called low-lethality method. The implication is that a low-lethality self-injurious act should be dismissed as attention-seeking. This is a myth – every suicidal act ought to be taken seriously; we should not infer lack of suicidal intent from the perceived lethality of a suicide attempt. Sometimes people think that self-cutting is less lethal than drug overdose. Indeed, I, like many others, used to be of the view that those who presented to hospital following a drug overdose were more likely to die by suicide in the future than those who presented following an episode of self-cutting. That was until Keith Hawton from the University of Oxford and his colleagues published a study showing the opposite. Using data from the Multicentre Study of Self-harm in England, they found that, among individuals aged 10–18 years, those who presented to hospital with self-cutting were more likely to die by suicide in the next few years than those who had been treated in hospital following an overdose.[25] In short, the take-home message is: every suicidal act or act of self-harm should be taken seriously.

# Part 2

# Suicide Is More About Ending the Pain Than Wanting To Die

It can be difficult to imagine ourselves in the shoes of others who are acutely suicidal. Even after all these years studying suicide, I have days when I find the personal cost of suicide completely bewildering and I worry about those who battle to stay alive. But even in these most difficult of moments, I try not to lose sight of the fact that suicide is driven by mental pain. Irrespective of its complex causes, suicide is about ending unbearable pain, albeit in a permanent way.

# 4

# Making Sense of a Suicide

WHEN FAMILIES OR grieving loved ones get in touch, they often want to know why. Why did their loved one take their own life? Why did they not see it coming or, if they did, why were they unable to prevent their loss? These emails, these letters, these telephone calls, are all stories of lost lives, the pain of brothers, sisters, mothers, fathers, friends, of sons and daughters, so personal and unique, but often so similar. Some are still in shock, devastated by loss, while others are angry or confused. All are at their wits' end, trying to make sense of their tragedy. These contacts usually come out of the blue; they may have found my name after an Internet search, heard me give a talk about suicide or read an academic paper of mine.

I was in my late twenties the first time I received such correspondence and I was pretty stumped initially, not sure how to respond. It was a handwritten letter, sent to my university address, asking whether I could telephone them. 'Them' were parents, parents to Daniel, whom they had lost just a few weeks before, who had no history of depression. Daniel was their only child, and his death came out of the blue and was 'completely out of character'. There was no email address, just a telephone number. They had come across something I had written that had resonated with them, so they had got in touch.

It was the year 2000, I would have been 27 and I was really struggling with imposter syndrome at the time. I was only a couple of years into my first lectureship, and I was still trying to establish myself as an independent researcher. As any new university lecturer can attest, you are often thrown into the deep end, struggling to keep one step ahead of the students. Certainly at that time, I didn't feel like I had a foothold in the suicide prevention research world. I was clearly still a novice, having only published my PhD work at that stage. 'What do I really know about understanding suicidal behaviour?', 'I have only been researching suicide for a wet weekend', 'They'd be better off speaking to someone else' . . . Such self-critical thoughts were on repeat in my head.

Unsurprisingly, therefore, I was hesitant about responding to the letter. I was genuinely flummoxed, in part because I was already feeling out of my depth. I didn't know what I would say and I was especially anxious that I would say the wrong thing or that I'd make their grief worse. Also, I didn't know how, in practical terms, making the actual telephone call would work. When would be a good time to phone? What should I say if they answered? How could I check that they were comfortable to speak? I role-played the call several times, but I just wasn't happy so I held off responding for a few days, trying to figure out how best to reply. I also didn't know how to communicate the boundaries of the call without appearing insensitive. I am not a therapist, I am a researcher and, without ever having met Daniel, I could never tell his parents why he had made the ultimate decision to take his own life. My concerns were similar to those of anyone who is broaching the subject of suicide with someone they don't necessarily know very well – I was concerned that I would say something that would make matters worse.

Even then, though, I had met enough people bereaved by suicide to know that by just having the opportunity to talk about their loved one, having the possibility of even the tiniest of glimpses into the darkness of the suicidal mind, can be helpful. As human beings we find it difficult to tolerate uncertainty or unknowns or ambiguities, we spend our lives trying to reduce them. From the minute we get up in the morning until we go to bed at night, we are striving to reduce these uncertainties and unknowns. Not only is suicide characterised by countless unknowns, but also by many unknowables. Unbearably, the one certainty about suicide, the one known, is that your loved one has gone and that they're not coming back. Never. Ever. Everything else is uncertain, confusing and complex. It is impossible to know what was going through someone's mind in those final minutes. Did they change their mind but it was too late? Did they think that no one cared about them? These are truly awful questions, but the reality is that the state of mind of those who have died at that moment of decision is unknowable.

That weekend I reasoned that my call could give the family an opportunity to 'test out' why they thought their loved one had died. Perhaps it could relieve a little of the uncertainty and provide a safe space for them to speak. The search for answers following a suicide is the most awful of paradoxes. The outcome is so definite, but the causes, the minutes or hours before death are so often hidden, but all-consuming for the bereaved. In 2008, when Clare died and I was faced with my own personal loss to suicide for the first time, I remembered this early encounter and how the pursuit for answers becomes so overwhelming, intractable and painful. All that you want more than anything else in the world is to have even five minutes with your loved one to ask them why they could not keep going, why they could not face living. You replay all of those past conversations, tormenting yourself about what you could or should have done to make things better. What you could or should have done to keep them alive. For days I scoured every single email I had received from Clare along with my replies to see how I could have responded differently.

I need not have worried about the call, about saying or doing the wrong thing. Both parents were at home when I rang the following week. They were in utter despair; traumatised, heartbroken and numb. They had barely ventured out of their home since Daniel's death. Rather they had been replaying his life, every significant milestone, every success and failure. There was no suicide note and, although he had no history of depression, he had been a casualty of the recession in the early nineties, losing his 'dream job' in 1991. His mother, in particular, thought he had never been the same after that. He was in his early thirties when he died and, in the three years before his death, he had lost another two jobs as well as his long-term relationship. He had begun to drink heavily and, according to his mother, had become a shadow of his former self. But he had never uttered anything about being hopeless or suicidal; he had been quite sanguine about the future so they had not been unduly concerned. Then, one evening, when they returned from dinner with friends, they found him. Lifeless. Like so many families, they could not pinpoint a specific final trigger or the 'straw that broke the camel's back'.

They had been at a loss to understand why and why then. Through their own meaning-making in the few weeks since his death, they had concluded that he had found moving back into the family home humiliating and he just couldn't see any other way to get his independence back. During the call, I mostly listened and tried to answer their questions as best I could, but in generalities; that most people in the UK who die by suicide are suffering from a mental health problem that can cloud their decision-making; that comorbidities, like problem alcohol use, can exacerbate existing mental health symptoms because alcohol is a depressant.[1] Daniel's parents found the idea of what psychologists call 'cognitive constriction' useful to understand why he may not have been able to see alternatives; seeing suicide as the only option for him. Cognitive constriction is often also referred to as tunnel vision – and this tunnel vision is such a common way of thinking in people who are suicidal.[2] Edwin Shneidman identified cognitive constriction as one of the common features of the suicidal mind many years ago, and treating this constriction is an important part of cognitive behavioural therapy (CBT), the widely used psychological treatment for common mental health problems including anxiety and depression as well people who are suicidal (see page 216).

When I first heard the term tunnel vision in a psychological context, it brought back a frightening memory from my childhood that I sometimes use to communicate what we mean by cognitive constriction, in part because it involves a tunnel! Close to my parents' house where I grew up in Derry in Northern Ireland, there was a place that was like a child's play paradise. It was a field with football pitches, fences and overgrown land, brilliant trees to climb and a stream. Quite a distance along the stream there was a tunnel. The details are pretty hazy all these years later, but I remember one winter's day when I was 10 or 11, I decided to run through the tunnel, but I fell over into the icy cold water and twisted my ankle. I was absolutely soaking wet and I didn't know where my friends had gone. I was alone and, despite shouting out, no one came. To make matters worse, it was dusk and I was unable to see the tunnel's exit. In my shocked state I couldn't think straight, my thinking just narrowed and narrowed, and all I could focus on was 'I am going to be stuck in this tunnel'. Even though I knew the tunnel had an end, I had never ventured that far before. Also, I didn't have the presence of mind to simply turn on my heel and hobble out. I felt physically stuck and I was also mentally stuck. I just couldn't think of a way to get out of the tunnel; my thinking was blinkered. Of course, my experience of being temporarily trapped in a wet, dark tunnel is nothing like the psychological pain associated with suicide, but it still gives an insight into how the mind can misconstrue events and situations and make us feel stuck, even when we may not be. On that occasion, despite a solution being possible, I couldn't think of a way out.

Sticking with this metaphor, suicidal thinking can be tunnel-like for several reasons; for some it is not possible to see the light at the end of the tunnel and for others it is like a mental trap, a cognitive prison from which they cannot escape. Whereas my childhood experience was temporary and I was able to escape my physical tunnel (when my friends eventually heard me call for help, they got one of the older kids to help me out), imagine what it feels like if you are trying to escape mental pain and your thinking just keeps getting narrower and narrower, more and more constricted. It is similar to being in a psychological tunnel where, in your mind, there is no way out. This way of thinking can be exhausting and it makes it difficult to see alternatives, to see a different future or a time when the mental pain will end.

Take 42-year-old Peter, for example, who took part in one of our research studies a few years ago, led by clinical psychologist Laura McDermott, on understanding the suicidal process.[3] He had a history of recurrent depression and he talked about the narrowing of focus that led to his suicide attempt:

> You lose your capacity to reason and rationalise and you just begin to focus on this desperate situation and how awful it is. At those times, you can't rationalise and say to yourself, 'You know what? Maybe tomorrow you can phone your GP or psychiatrist or Samaritans.'

In that interview, Peter also talked about his desperation and sense of powerlessness:

> Over the years as my depression has got worse and it has been a more long-term experience, I think the suicide attempts, when I have felt suicidal, that feeling has been more intense. You think, 'I am back at this point again. I have felt like this so many times in the past. I have tried but nothing works.' So I think when it happens, there is more desperation and just wanting it to really work this time. It's a bit like you keep trying something and trying something and want it to work. You become more desperate for it to work.

People who are suicidal often feel like no one else can hear them or feel their pain and they cannot see another way out. Like me being in the actual tunnel all those years ago, it seemed to me that no matter how loud I shouted all I could hear was my own echo.

Here is Annie, a 32-year-old woman whom Laura interviewed as part of the same study. She had attempted suicide on several occasions and had a history of major depressive disorder and post-traumatic stress disorder. In this part of the interview she talks about how she just couldn't continue:

> I just remember it feeling like the straw that broke the camel's back and I just thought, 'I can't do this. I can't keep trying to fit in this world. I can't keep trying to persevere and maintain a presence. It is not possible for me anymore.' And that is when I took an overdose.

Peter and Annie give us some insight into the patterns of thinking associated with suicide. Their comments highlight the often unrelenting nature of the struggle to stay alive. I will return to such struggles later.

### Shame and anger

Not all such telephone calls or meetings have gone as smoothly over the years as the one with Daniel's parents did. Not that long ago, I met with a mother, Shilpa, who had lost her seventeen-year-old daughter Kiara six months before. She was a friend of a friend and I knew some of the details in advance, mainly through media reports of the tragedy. We met face-to-face and, although I still don't quite understand how I didn't see it coming, halfway through our conversation something I said triggered Shilpa, and she became very upset. Becoming upset is not that surprising, but it was the intensity of the anger and rage that took me aback. The details of the conversation were not that different from many others that I have regularly: Shilpa was angry, with the school, with child and adolescent mental health services and with Kiara. We talked about the circumstances leading up to the death; Kiara had a history of self-harm and depression, she had been bullied and had issues around eating from puberty onwards. Even at such a young age, according to her mother, she had had enough, none of the treatments she had received had worked and she was relieved, in part, that Kiara was no longer suffering. But she was so conflicted; like so many bereaved family members, she just could not come to terms with the pain that Kiara had inflicted on the family. She felt that Kiara had been selfish in taking her life. And then, at the same time, she felt so guilty, sick to the pit of her stomach guilty, for thinking so badly of her daughter.

We had a wide-ranging conversation about adolescent self-harm that afternoon, about the myriad factors that contribute to self-harm, and self-harm's relationship with suicide.[4] We talked about whether suicide was a selfish act or not. I told her that I didn't think it was selfish and I focused on the evidence that when someone is suicidal, struggling with thoughts of whether to live or die, they are usually not able to see the pain that their death would cause to others. I reiterated that, counterintuitively, they often feel that they are relieving their loved ones of a burden.[5] As soon as I uttered the word 'burden', Shilpa's anger became apparent. It transpired that, although she had thought she had 'come to terms' with Kiara's death and understood the mental pain that had driven her daughter to suicide, her anger was focused on the pain the death had caused her family – that the family was broken and it would never be the same again. She said over and over that Kiara was selfish and that she was ashamed of her daughter while also feeling ashamed of herself for thinking such thoughts. It was like a triple whammy of shame, anger and guilt, with shame and anger directed both at herself and her daughter. Again, without talking about the specifics around Kiara's life, I tried to explain how, from a psychological perspective, people who are suicidal see the world – especially how they perceive their future through a lens that is blinkered and clouded with unrelenting pessimism – and that Kiara may have been so mentally exhausted that she could not see or appreciate the pain that her death would cause.[6]

When Shilpa left, I didn't know what to think. The conversation ended amicably, but I didn't feel that I had connected with her, or that she had found what I had said helpful. However, some months after our meeting, she got back in touch. It was ostensibly to apologise for breaking down when we met, but also to tell me that she was now seeing a psychologist who was really helping her through her loss, and this was helping her to make sense of the relationship she had with Kiara in life and also the relationship she now had with her and their shared memories. She also said that her anger had subsided, that it still came in waves, but that she no longer erupts with rage. She also added that, although she couldn't make sense of the 'psychological perspective' when we met, it had helped her to think differently about the mental torture that Kiara must have experienced for so long before her death.

Like so many people bereaved by suicide whom I have met over the years, I have struggled with the very same 'why' questions myself when I have been faced with my own personal encounters with suicide bereavement, first Clare in 2008, and then Noel in 2011. And although I am still striving to find answers, well over a decade later, I appreciate the importance of being able to ask these questions – and I am keen to help others similarly bereaved, if I can. Sadly though, none of us can truly answer the why questions, so what I try to do now is to bring to bear my 25 years of experience working in suicide research and prevention to understand something of each individual, and their unique and valued life. I make it clear, but I hope I do so with compassion, that I cannot give family members or friends the answers they so badly need. I cannot tell them why their son, daughter, another relative or friend took their own life. But by explaining what I have learned about the complex causes of suicide, I hope I can provide some insight that may help them make sense of their own loss. By recounting my experiences of talking to others about their loss in this book, I hope it's evident that, as long as we do so with compassion and sensitivity, we are unlikely to say the wrong thing. My advice is, if in doubt, please reach out and connect. We should never underestimate the power of human connection.

# 5

# What Suicide Is Not

MOST PEOPLE WHO lose a loved one to suicide have never thought about the causes of suicide before tragedy comes knocking. All they may know about suicide is what they have read in a book or have heard in the media. As I noted in Chapter 3, myths and misinformation abound about suicide, so before we explore any further what drives someone to suicide, let's think about what suicide is not.

## Suicide is not selfish

Characterising suicide as selfish simply adds to the stigma around it. And when stigma increases, help-seeking declines, ignorance flourishes and deaths soar. Daniel and Kiara, who we met in the previous chapter, were not selfish, they were in pain, and suicide was their means of ending that pain. In their different ways, their deaths were acts of desperation. If you have never been in that dark place, it can be difficult not to see suicide as anything other than selfish. But the reality is that, for the vast majority of people, they see their suicide as a selfless act, their way of trying to stop the suffering that they perceive they are causing their loved ones.[1]

## Suicide is not the coward's way out

This phrase has a long history in the discourse around suicide, but again, it is unhelpful, stigmatising and insulting to many. When people suggest that suicide is cowardly, I usually ask them to think about what they understand by the meaning of coward, to consider the individual words that may trip too easily off their tongues. Irrespective of the method of suicide, to end one's life is difficult. Not only do you have to overcome the most basic self-preservation instinct, but for many the act of ending one's life is physically painful. It is most definitely not a cowardly act; it is an act of desperation and most often a manifestation of unbearable mental pain.

## Suicide is not caused by a single factor

Like any other cause of death, the factors that lead to suicide are multiple and varied. However, too often the media representations of suicide are simplistic. For example, newspaper headlines such as 'Cyberbullying killed my son' used to be quite common, but thankfully as more and more media outlets adhere to the reporting guidelines, such irresponsible reporting has declined.[2]

In the same way that smoking is one of the risk factors for death from lung cancer, we also know that a range of other genetic, clinical, psychosocial and cultural factors play a role. Suicide is no different in this regard from other causes of death – there is no single risk factor; there are many pathways to suicide involving multiple risk factors.[3]

## Suicide is not explained by mental illness

I wrote about the parallels between preventing cancer and tackling suicide in one of my first research articles in 1999 for *Health Psychology Update*, the newsletter of the British Psychological Society's Division of Health Psychology.[4] In addition to highlighting that suicide was not caused by a single factor, it was the first time I suggested that suicide should be thought of as a health behaviour in the same way that smoking is as a risk factor for cancer. This may strike you as an incidental or obvious point, but it was linked to a nagging concern I had that suicide was too often explained as a by-product of mental illness. As a consequence, it wasn't seen as an entity, a thing, a behaviour, in its own right. I always considered this to be unhelpful, because although suicide and mental illness often co-occur, the presence of mental illness does not explain why an individual attempts or dies by suicide. I have lost count of the number of times, in response to the question, 'Why did so and so kill themselves?', the answer given is 'because they were depressed'. Depression may have been part of the landscape surrounding many people's deaths by suicide, but it does not explain why someone ends their life. Indeed, fewer than 5 per cent of those who are treated in hospital for depression – the mental illness most commonly associated with suicide – go on to kill themselves.[5] This view is also linked to the stigmatising myth that suicide is an abnormal act carried out by people who are 'mad'. The corollary of this is that if the act is abnormal and the person who engages in such behaviour is mad, then it is inexplicable and therefore it cannot be prevented. This is utter rubbish!

As a health psychologist, conceptualising suicide as a behaviour is significant because it opens up a whole range of potential avenues in terms of understanding and preventing suicide. In the 1999 paper mentioned above, I described suicidal behaviour as the 'ultimate health-jeopardising behaviour'. To put this in context, when I started my research career, suicide was firmly located within the domains of clinical psychology and psychiatry. Although this was understandable, I thought this was misguided and that advances in understanding and treating suicidal thoughts and behaviours were being hampered as a result. The main concern I had was that, at that time, mental illness explanations for suicide were dominant and they didn't take into sufficient consideration the psychological and social determinants of suicide. Neither clinical psychology nor psychiatry, as mental health disciplines, really considered suicide to be a behaviour whereas, to my mind, this was blindingly obvious. So my mantra since then has been that suicide is first and foremost a behaviour; it is something that someone does. If we treat it as a behaviour and target suicidal thoughts and behaviours directly as intervention targets, we are likely to have more success in preventing suicide. Embracing health psychology and all that it can offer alongside the other disciplines allows us to do the former and much more comprehensively.

As a scientific discipline, health psychology has traditionally focused on physical health, illness, healthcare and well-being to the exclusion of mental health. This exclusion has always felt arbitrary to me, and it grew out of turf wars between clinical psychology (the sub-discipline of psychology focused on mental health) and the newer discipline of health psychology (or medical psychology) in the eighties. As it happens, a couple of years ago, I was interviewed as part of an oral history of the development of health psychology in the UK.[6] This was an interesting experience and, as part of this, I reflected upon the reality that my work on suicide was definitely seen as being at the margins of health psychology in the nineties. Thankfully, this has changed considerably since. Indeed in recent years, I have been honoured to deliver keynote addresses at the leading health psychology conferences in the UK and Europe. One of the hallmarks of health psychology relevant to suicide prevention is that it has at its disposal a whole range of theoretical models that were developed specifically to predict health behaviours. When I was starting out, a group of models called the 'social cognition models' were dominant in health psychology. Social cognition models try to predict behaviour from a range of beliefs and attitudes that capture internal (cognitive) and social processes hypothesised to govern behaviour. Over the years, these models have been used extensively and with considerable success to predict a myriad of health behaviours including smoking, drinking, adherence to medication and help-seeking.[7]

Up until the early noughties though, social cognition models had been rarely applied to mental health and had never been applied to predicting suicidal behaviour. Indeed, at a health psychology conference in 1999 (which led me to write the article for *Health Psychology Update*) I suggested to a colleague that we should harness social cognition models to understand suicidal behaviour, but he was immediately dismissive. His argument was that suicide is caused by mental illness, people who are mentally ill are abnormal, and if they are abnormal it isn't possible to apply psychological models of so-called 'normal' behaviour to understanding and predicting suicide. I was surprised by this standpoint, but it succinctly illustrated in one encounter the implicit stigma around suicide as well as a misunderstanding of mental illness.

According to this view, if you have a mental illness then, for some unknown reason, the rules that govern your behaviour are different from those that govern the behaviour of those without a mental illness. It is dehumanising and, although it has its roots in fear and ignorance, it is highly stigmatising, not to mention incorrect. This is another good example of 'othering' – rather than seeing mental health on a continuum, it falls into the trap of treating people who struggle with mental health problems as being qualitatively different from those who don't. We all have mental health and we are all somewhere along the mental health–mental ill health continuum, with those of us who are more fortunate being somewhere towards the end that doesn't involve mental anguish.

## Suicide is not a sin

As someone who grew up in Ireland I was aware of the damage that Catholic teaching on suicide did to many families the length and breadth of the country. Up until the eighties, people who died by suicide were often not afforded the common decency of a burial on the so-called hallowed ground of a church. It took a papal decree to reverse the Church's official position in 1983, allowing Catholic families to bury their loved ones regardless of cause of death. More than a decade after this decree, the impact of such religious teachings on some families was made pretty clear to me. After my first appearance on TV towards the end of my PhD in the mid-nineties – a local news item about one of my research studies – out of the blue, I received a letter from a family who lived in a rural part of Northern Ireland. They wanted to share their story about the loss of their son to suicide, who had died after a long struggle with mental health problems. They wished me well with my research and they were keen to help, if they could. It was a really moving letter, littered with guilt and shame, so much so that the sentiments remain with me still today. Sadly, the parents were of that generation where suicide deaths were not always accorded a proper Church burial and their correspondence is likely a product of their era. Nonetheless, their words, handwritten, were heartbreaking. In addition to feeling that they had failed their son and that they should have done more, they were also of the firm belief that they had brought shame on the Church and on their local community. In their eyes, their son had committed a mortal sin, and this was unforgivable. However, they didn't blame their son, they blamed themselves. This really angered me, not anger towards them, rather anger towards the Church. Instead of providing solace in their hour of need, the legacy of the Church's teachings was detrimental, isolating them from their faith and their community. Thankfully, things have moved on and I have seen, at first hand, countless times, the incredible work that churches do and how important religion is for so many people bereaved by suicide.

Also, it wasn't until 2015 that the General Synod of the Church of England updated the sixteenth-century *Book of Common Prayer*, which stated that a funeral service may not be used 'for any that . . . have laid violent hands upon themselves'. In many parts of the world, suicide is still considered a sin and, in some, a criminal act. Suicide is illegal in at least 25 countries and attempted suicide is punishable under Sharia law in a further 10. Such attitudes and laws are outdated and wrong, causing needless suffering to millions of people across the globe. I am proud to be the President of the IASP, which advocates in these countries for the decriminalisation of suicidal behaviour.[8] But we can all play our part by lobbying political and religious representatives in countries in which suicide remains a crime.

## Suicide is not the fault of those bereaved

It is important to remember that the suicide of your loved one is not your fault. Sadly, and all too often, those left behind, those bereaved by suicide, blame themselves, thinking that they should have done more. The guilt and regret can be especially painful if the last encounter they had with their loved one was an argument or a disagreement. Unfortunately, it is likely that an interpersonal crisis such as an argument will have occurred in the hours, days or weeks before the death. When I think back to my first published academic paper, a detailed examination of the factors associated with 142 suicides in Belfast, Northern Ireland, we found that marital or relationship problems were the most frequently reported stressor.[9] But this does not imply causality and, as I have said time and again, suicide is caused by multiple factors. In addition, no one would ever expect an argument or disagreement to end in the death of their loved one. Irrespective of the circumstances, a single individual should never be held responsible for another person's actions.

The common theme running through each of these *nots* is that suicide is driven by the desire to end one's pain rather than wanting to die. The causes of suicide are complex and we need to look beyond mental illness explanations to understand why 800,000 people lose their lives to suicide each year. In the next few chapters, I will do just that by guiding you through the model of suicide that I developed, which I hope will help you understand how mental pain emerges to increase suicide risk.

# Towards An Integrated Understanding of Suicide

DURING THE SUMMER months of 2010, I was preoccupied with finalising the first edition of *The International Handbook of Suicide Prevention* that I was co-editing with my colleagues Steve Platt and Jacki Gordon – feeling under pressure because the publisher's deadline for delivery of the final manuscript was fast approaching.[1] The idea for the handbook had grown out of a European conference on suicide and suicidal behaviour that Steve, Jacki and I had organised in 2008. I was delighted to be working with Steve, because it was some of his seminal research on unemployment and suicide that had inspired me back in the nineties at Queen's.[2] It was also a delight to work with Jacki, who brought the government policy expertise to the book. We invited all of our keynote speakers from the conference plus other experts from across the world to contribute chapters on hot topics in suicide research and prevention.

When we had signed the book contract, I had put myself down to deliver a chapter on the 'psychology of suicide', without giving much thought to its content or structure. Then, not long before the submission deadline, I set about writing my chapter. But it felt like such a fruitless task, as I couldn't get much beyond a few pages, dryly summarising some of our latest research on understanding suicide and self-harm. After a few more unproductive days persevering with the writing, I decided to abandon my 'here-are-all-of-the-psychological-factors-associated-with-suicide' plan for the chapter and replace it with something on a new theoretical model focused on understanding suicide. I was keen to do so as a means of integrating the diverse range of risk and protective factors into a single overarching framework. Developing such a model had been something I had been mulling over for some time by then as I was keen to distil my thinking about what I had learned in the previous 10–15 years of working in the field of suicide research.

My aim was to develop a model that better described the complex processes that lead people to become suicidal in the first place and, crucially, to map out the factors that govern the transition from thinking about ending one's life to attempting to do so. To my mind, getting to grips with this transition is one of the Holy Grails in suicide prevention research (others include developing tailored psychological treatments that are effective in reducing suicide risk and improving our ability to predict suicide with an acceptable degree of accuracy). I hoped that the model would help to elucidate why people become suicidal in the first place and why some people act on their thoughts of suicide and others do not. I also wanted it to provide a framework on which treatment interventions could be developed. Moreover, I wanted to create a model that looked beyond mental illness to map out the pathways to suicidal thinking and behaviour.

## Suicide, Escape and Entrapment

After a slow start, I found the writing process liberating and within a couple of weeks it resulted in the integrated motivational–volitional (IMV) model of suicidal behaviour (which we'll explore in detail in the next chapter).[3] To get there, I reread countless academic papers and books on suicide that I hadn't looked at for years, going back to Edwin Shneidman and Norman Farberow's seminal 1957 book, *Clues to Suicide*, and Shneidman's 1967 *Essays in Self-destruction*, as well as other influential research, such as a theoretical paper entitled 'Suicide as escape from self' by the social psychologist Roy Baumeister.[4] Published in 1990, drawing on different historical and theoretical perspectives, Baumeister's paper argued persuasively that the primary motivation for suicide was escape. He wasn't the first person to propose an escape theory of suicide. In the seventies, Jean Baechler had proposed a taxonomy of suicide that included escape as one category and others such as Shneidman had previously recognised the importance of escape.[5] However, what Baumeister did that caught my attention was distil the key elements of previous theoretical efforts in a way that was intuitively appealing as well as being grounded within the scientific method.

When I first read Baumeister's paper in the early days of my PhD, I was left with more questions than answers (a good thing in my opinion), but his core idea of suicide being a means of escaping yourself really resonated with me. It just made sense. And it has been central to my research ever since. So much so that I sometimes question how much my thinking has actually evolved in the intervening 20 years. Baumeister had also built upon Shneidman's earlier thinking, and Baumeister's work, in turn, was extended by the Oxford clinical psychologist and pioneer in mindfulness research, Mark Williams. As academic inspirations go, for me they don't get any more influential than Mark Williams. Not only did he conduct innovative research into the suicidal mind, but he also developed groundbreaking psychological treatments and has the uncanny ability to communicate the most complex of ideas with such ease and warmth. Indeed, it was he who introduced me to the concept of 'suicidal entrapment' in his classic *Cry of Pain* that was published in 1997, the year I completed my PhD.[6] His framing of suicide as a 'cry of pain' rather than as a 'cry for help' was also important in highlighting the human face of the distress that underpins suicide, as well as challenging the stigma around it.

According to Williams, suicide is an escape from entrapment. I know that sounds a bit like an oxymoron, but let me try to explain. According to the *Oxford English Dictionary*, entrapment 'is the state of being caught in or as in a trap'. In other words, you're caught in a situation from which there is no way out. Paul Gilbert, a British clinical psychologist who did a lot of the early theoretical work on the role of entrapment in mental distress, talks about entrapment as occurring when one's desire to flee from an unpleasant situation (usually a defeating or humiliating situation) is blocked.[7] His thinking was influenced by evolutionary theory. The debilitating consequences associated with not being able to escape from unwanted situations were first documented in animals, not in humans. Indeed, many years ago, ethologists observed that if an animal is defeated in, say, a fight with another animal and it is not able to escape from that defeating or humiliating situation, it can often end up being helpless.[8] They labelled this situation 'arrested flight', as the animal's attempt to flee is blocked; and it is this entrapment rather than the defeat or humiliation that is so pernicious in the human as well as the animal context. Whereas entrapment was initially used by Paul Gilbert as a means of understanding human depression, Mark Williams extended its application to suicide risk, specifically. In short, therefore, suicidal behaviour is an attempt to escape from being trapped by mental pain.

Entrapment can be assessed in different ways, but the most widely used measure is the Entrapment Scale developed by Paul Gilbert and Steven Allan in 1998.[9] This is a 16-item self-report scale that assesses overall entrapment as well as internal and external entrapment. Internal entrapment is feeling trapped by unbearable thoughts and feelings, whereas external entrapment is when the feelings of entrapment are driven by defeating or humiliating circumstances. And suicidal thoughts emerge when efforts to escape these thoughts and feelings are thwarted. People are asked to indicate on a five-point scale the extent to which each item (e.g., 'I feel trapped inside myself') applies to them (from 'not at all like me' to 'extremely like me') and the higher the score, the more trapped they are. In our clinical studies we often use the Entrapment Scale to tap the levels of entrapment shortly after a suicide attempt to see whether the responses help us to understand who is most at risk of future suicidal behaviour.

In one of our studies published in 2013 with Mark Williams, we asked a group of patients who had been admitted to hospital following a suicide attempt to complete a range of psychological and clinical measures including measures of depression, hopelessness, entrapment and current levels of suicidal ideation.[10] Using data linkage and with the patients' permission we were able to track who attempted suicide again or who sadly died by suicide over the next four years. This allowed us to determine which of the factors that we had assessed in the hospital four years before predicted future suicide risk. These findings were important, because although depression and suicidal ideation predicted future suicidal behaviour, the best predictors of suicidal behaviour were levels of entrapment and past history of suicidal behaviour. Evidently, it is not possible to do anything about someone's suicidal history. However, it might be possible to target and possibly change their levels of entrapment. Therefore, if we can reduce how trapped someone feels, we can potentially break the link between entrapment and suicide risk. Other studies involving thousands of participants across a range of different populations, including young people and general population samples, have also found a strong association between entrapment and suicidal thoughts and attempts – the more trapped the person feels, the more likely they are to have suicidal thoughts and make attempts to end their own lives.[11] I firmly believe that entrapment is key to understanding the suicidal mind.

Most often in our research, we have used the original 16-item Entrapment Scale, but together with Dutch psychologist Derek de Beurs, we published the four-item Entrapment Short-Form (E-SF) in 2020.[12] This short-form questionnaire has the pragmatic advantage of taking less time to complete; therefore it is easier to integrate into everyday clinical practice or research studies. The first two statements assess external entrapment and the final two assess internal entrapment. If time or space is really tight, only asking people about the two internal entrapment statements works pretty well also.

1. I often have the feeling that I would just like to run away.
2. I feel powerless to change things.

3. I feel trapped inside myself.
4. I feel I'm in a deep hole I can't get out of.

In the studies that we and other research groups have conducted, internal entrapment appears to be much more dangerous than external entrapment. For example, in one of our studies, led by Karen Wetherall, we found that internal entrapment predicted suicidal ideation over 12 months in young people.[13] It is interesting to pause for a minute to think about why this might be. Clearly internal and external entrapment are intricately linked, but it's the need to escape one's thoughts or feelings that seems to become so unbearable. Of course, what's going on in our heads is so often driven by external circumstances, but in terms of the central drivers of suicidal thinking, these are so often internal. It can be difficult for others to see these thoughts and feelings because they are intangible and ethereal, but despite not being visible, they are *more* not less painful.

A few years ago I had a conversation with Ed, who had attempted suicide in his thirties, and we discussed this very issue of different types of entrapment. He had just turned 40 when we spoke and he was in reflective mode, trying to make sense of the highs and lows of his life. The idea of internal versus external entrapment seemed to fit so well with what happened to him. He felt that being externally trapped – his marriage had broken down and he was no longer able to see his children – preceded his feelings of internal entrapment. After the break-up, he felt completely worthless and abandoned. These feelings of internal entrapment escalated and escalated, pervading other aspects of his life, so that his self-critical thoughts seemed to be never-ending. Although he recognised that the consequences of the marriage breakdown were only part of why he became suicidal, he was exhausted, and it was the non-stop negative thoughts that he tried to extinguish when he attempted suicide.

As Ed's story illustrates, internal entrapment conjures up images of being out of control and helpless. For me, and I imagine countless others, when the going gets tough, I gain incredible solace from retreating into myself, taking comfort in my own thoughts and recalling past images and events that have brought me pleasure and happiness. I metaphorically fill myself up on these pleasant memories and fantasies. My mind is my safe space. However, the difficulty arises when one feels trapped internally, when our internal world becomes a source of pain rather than of comfort. It no longer feels like a safe space. And if this pain and perceived lack of safety escalate, a bit like a storm brewing, then it can begin to feel more and more like there is nowhere safe to hide, nowhere to rest or relax, nowhere left to escape to because existentially you are trying to escape yourself. At such times, suicidal thoughts are much more likely to erupt because, in such a trapped state, we find it impossible to imagine a time when these thoughts will subside. We become imprisoned by our thoughts and feelings. We are trapped inside ourselves and feel that there is no escape. And it's exhausting. If we add into the mix that these thoughts are often contaminated by feelings of shame, loss, self-hate, rejection and anger, we can begin to get a sense of what mental pain feels like.

## Mental Pain

Entrapment is mental pain and mental pain can be entrapping. When in mental pain we search for solutions to end that pain;

this search may include distracting oneself from the pain, talking to family or friends, removing oneself from the defeating situation, taking medication, drinking alcohol to dull the pain, seeking professional help, or countless other things to help cope with or manage the pain. Sadly though, as entrapment increases and if no solutions are found, the likelihood that we consider suicide as a means of escape increases. This is when tunnel vision can make things precarious, because the more blinkered we are in our thinking, the fewer and fewer potential solutions come to mind. As each potential solution is discounted or dismissed, we edge another step closer to concluding that suicide is *the* solution – the ultimate but permanent solution to ending the pain. The rate at which the discounting happens is different for each of us. As a result, for some, the suicidal act may appear impulsive and for others it may seem to be more measured. Clearly, for most of us, suicide is never the conclusion we come to when we experience mental pain.

Similarly, mental pain can take many different forms. Some people, like Ed, describe the pain in terms of needing the seemingly relentless thinking to end; that the turmoil in their heads is exhausting. They may be overwhelmed by a never-ending ruminative cycle of negative thoughts about themselves, the world and their future – or, more commonly, their lack of a future.[14] Humza, a 26-year-old man who spoke to us about a previous suicide attempt for one of our interview studies, made this point quite succinctly: 'I just wanted to stop thinking about everything . . . I gave up on life. I didn't particularly want to experience what the future might hold. I felt like I had humiliated my family and I just knew that no matter what I did, they'd never forgive me.' Humza could not cope with thinking; attempting suicide was his way of stopping himself from doing so.

Annie, whom we met earlier, who has attempted suicide a few times before, also sees suicidal behaviour as her only option, the only solution, a means of exercising control when all else has been taken away:

> It's sometimes the only option, the only power you have left in your life. Because life takes everything away from you. Your self-worth. Your achievements. Your community. Your friends. Your family. How you feel about yourself. Because when it is all gone, you will have a decision left and that is whether or not to live.

When I first read Annie's words, they reminded me of the oft-quoted lines from *The Myth of Sisyphus* by the Nobel Laureate Albert Camus, who mused that, '[T]here is but one truly serious philosophical problem, and that is suicide. Judging whether life is or is not worth living amounts to answering the fundamental question of philosophy.'[15] Sadly, though, in the moment of suicidal crisis, an individual's thinking is too often caught in a mental trap that clouds clear judgement. Despite Camus's eloquent prose, therefore, any thoughts about the future are not so much questions of philosophy, but more questions of how to escape.

Matt Haig, author of the bestselling memoir, *Reasons to Stay Alive*, recently posted about escape on Instagram, which fits well with what Baumeister outlined in his escape theory.[16] Matt notes that: 'There comes a beautiful point where you have to stop trying to escape yourself or improve yourself and just really accept yourself.' Although Matt wasn't referring to suicide, his sentence rings so true, and it relates directly to suicide risk, and it resonates with some of what Humza and Annie said.

The challenge, though, is how do we help ourselves, and others, to stop trying to escape themselves? Suicide often arises out of agitation, or is driven by a traumatic past, by regret or self-criticism, usually rooted in misguided self-hatred that contributes to mental pain that becomes unbearable. Sadly, for too many of us, it is so difficult to do as Haig says, and accept ourselves.

Haig's Instagram post wasn't his first foray into talking about escape or entrapment. I had the pleasure of taking part in two literary events with Matt when *Reasons to Stay Alive* was first published in 2015. The book describes his descent into suicidal crisis when he was 24 and what he has learned since about living better and staying alive. It is a great read; moving, insightful and at times very funny. Without doubt, it has helped countless people navigate the depths of suicidal despair and find new meaning in life. For the first event, at the Edinburgh International Book Festival, I wanted to do something a little different. I was keen to use Haig's own words in *Reasons to Stay Alive* to illustrate what I had planned to say on the psychology of suicide. So, in preparation, I scoured his book, going through it line by line, searching for instances where Matt had talked about escape or entrapment in the context of his distress. I didn't have to look for too long before finding the first example – literally, on the first page, he describes being stuck. Indeed, I kept looking and kept finding references to escape and entrapment – they are recurrent themes throughout his book. If you haven't read Haig's book, I urge you to do so. It is life-affirming.

Of course, not every individual who feels trapped or is trying to escape themselves is consciously dismissing each potential solution one by one. However, they are likely to be going through some type of process of elimination, trying to find a way through their pain. To make matters worse, this process can be 'short-cutted' if, for example, they are drinking alcohol or taking drugs or they have been unable to sleep. Alcohol researchers often talk about 'alcohol myopia', the idea that when we drink, we become short-sighted, not being able to see the longer-term consequences of our actions.[17] This myopia renders it less likely that we can see alternative solutions, less able to recognise that there will be a time in the future when the pain will end. As a consequence, the discounting process becomes accelerated, making it more likely that suicide emerges as *the* solution. It's a bit like a horse cantering, then galloping, gathering more and more speed as it goes and becoming less and less able to control as it gets faster and faster. Also, alcohol is disinhibiting, facilitating rash actions, making suicidal behaviour more and more inevitable with each unit we imbibe. The dangerous effects of alcohol really came through in a review that my colleagues, Cara Richardson and Katie Robb, and I conducted, where we found strong evidence for the role of alcohol problems in male suicide.[18]

I read Gail Honeyman's bestselling novel *Eleanor Oliphant is Completely Fine* recently and I was struck by her description of the protagonist Eleanor's suicide attempt.[19] Honeyman's narrative, recounting the hours before Eleanor's suicide attempt, is especially powerful – and sadly will be familiar to many. It painfully illustrates how alcohol disrupts our decision-making, exacerbates feelings of worthlessness and reduces our decisions to binary options, to 'either-ors', 'should I live or should I die?'. In the haze of an alcohol-fuelled suicidal crisis, it can be difficult, nigh on impossible, to see beyond the present, with the present and the future fused together in a seemingly never-ending vortex of pain and nothingness. But as Eleanor's story strikingly conveys, together with countless real-life examples, recovery is possible. In Eleanor's case, a friend intervenes in her moment of crisis. For others, it could be a serendipitous act that saves their life, or the support of a mental health professional, or a reconnection with a family member, or even an act of kindness from a stranger. Indeed, Ryan's story in Chapter 2 (see page 45) illustrates the power of small acts of kindness. Anything that increases one's options, no matter how brief, could help someone to find a way out of their darkness.

# The Integrated Motivational–Volitional Model of Suicidal Behaviour

IN THIS CHAPTER, I will help you to understand the pathways from mental pain to suicidal thoughts and from suicidal thoughts to acts of suicide. Suicidal thoughts and suicidal ideation have the same meaning and, therefore, are used interchangeably throughout. I will look beyond mental illness explanations of suicide and provide a detailed description of what factors to look out for if you are concerned that a loved one may be suicidal or at risk of acting on their thoughts of suicide. The integrated motivational–volitional (IMV) model will provide a framework to try to make sense of suicidality and help you understand why some people become suicidal in the first place and others may die by suicide.[1]

Before I describe the IMV model in more detail, it might be helpful to take a few minutes to familiarise yourself with Figure 1, while bearing in mind the following four points:

- The IMV model is more straightforward than it looks at first glance.
- Ignore the technical language for now (I'll unpick this as we go along).

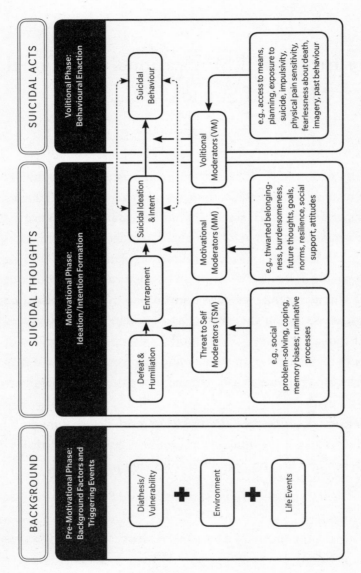

Figure 1. The integrated motivational–volitional model of suicidal behaviour[2]

- Entrapment acts like a bridge that links defeat and humiliation to suicidal ideation.
- The factors that lead to suicidal thoughts are different from those that lead to suicidal behaviour.

When I am describing the IMV model in talks, I tend to begin with the following key observations:

- The model is divided into three parts or phases as follows:

  1. Phase one covers the background context in which suicide risk may emerge (pre-motivational phase).
  2. Phase two focuses on the emergence of suicidal thoughts (motivational phase).
  3. Phase three maps out the factors that make suicidal acts more likely if someone is thinking about suicide (volitional phase).

My long-time friend and collaborator Ronan O'Carroll, a clinical and health psychologist, likes to describe the three phases of the model as vulnerability, motivation and action (VMA), respectively. And I have to admit that this is a very good short-hand description. Next, I usually provide some more detail about the emergence of suicidal thoughts/ideation versus suicidal behaviour:

- Suicidal ideation is more likely to emerge if you feel defeated or humiliated and, importantly, as though you cannot escape from these feelings. Feelings of entrapment – being trapped – are the key driver of suicidal ideation. Alongside defeat and humiliation, these feelings of entrapment are the fuel upon which suicidal ideation thrives. The defeat → entrapment → suicidal ideation → suicidal behaviour pathway is the backbone of the model.

- As I noted above, the factors leading to suicidal ideation are different from those that increase the likelihood that a person attempts suicide or dies by suicide. It isn't simply that people who are more suicidal are more likely to attempt suicide, rather that there is a distinct group of factors that appear to be particularly associated with suicidal acts rather than suicidal thoughts.

In the sections that follow I'll unpack each of these observations in more detail as I describe each phase in turn, but first I want to outline the principles that lie behind the model.

## Guiding Principles of the IMV Model

When I was developing the IMV model I had five guiding principles in mind, summarised below, that I hope help with understanding it and its application. First off, despite being embedded in the psychology of suicide, I wanted to put forward a model that could take account of the genetic, biological, social and cultural influences on suicide risk. I talk about these influences, such as early life trauma, later (see page 121). In essence, the model frames such influences as having their primary effect on suicide risk through their impact on the psychological factors within the motivational and volitional phases of the model. In particular, these influences and experiences increase suicide risk by affecting our perceptions of the past, the present and the future. Of course, the pathways to suicide are so much more than perceptions, but perceptions are central to understanding suicide risk as they are informed by our biology, our environment and our life experiences. And the decision to end one's life is driven by how we perceive our existence in terms of its present, its past and ultimately its future. Making the difficult decision to end one's life is not the same as an individual choosing to die. For most people, suicide is not a real choice as, for them, their life has become so unbearable that suicide is the only means of ending their mental pain.

Second, I wanted the model to build upon other theoretical models in the field of suicide research, hence my choice of name: the *integrated* motivational–volitional model. It would be a bit of a tangent to describe each of these models in turn, but if you're interested in learning more, they are outlined in *The International Handbook of Suicide Prevention*.[3] That said, three models are important to highlight. As I noted earlier, my thinking has been strongly influenced by Mark Williams' and Paul Gilbert's work on the cry of pain and the arrested flight models, respectively.[4] Their insights led directly to the inclusion of defeat and entrapment in the IMV model. The other model that has been influential is Thomas Joiner's Interpersonal Theory of Suicide (IPTS).[5] The IPTS, in its most parsimonious form, states that suicidal ideation (or suicidal desire, as Joiner describes it) emerges from the interplay of feeling a burden on others (perceived burdensomeness) and not feeling that you belong (thwarted belongingness). According to the IPTS, however, it is when a third factor – the capability for suicide – is present that a serious suicide attempt may occur. In Joiner's model, capability comprises two factors: fearlessness about death and physical pain tolerance. I'll return to these later, but in effect, capability for suicide is thought to change over time and, among those with suicidal desire, when fearlessness about dying is high and levels of physical pain tolerance are high, the risk of a suicidal act is increased.

Take another look at Figure 1 and you'll see that these factors are included within the motivational (defeat, entrapment, burdensomeness and belongingness) and volitional (physical pain sensitivity and fearlessness about death) phases of the IMV model. The motivational–volitional distinction speaks to the third principle, that the model should help us to better identify who will develop thoughts of suicide and who will act on their self-destructive thoughts.

The fourth principle that guided my thinking was that, from a scientific point of view, the model should generate specific questions and hypotheses that are directly testable in research studies. This is important because hypothesis testing is the cornerstone of science. We put forward hypotheses and then we gather data to see whether the hypotheses are supported or not. If they are not, then we need to think again, perhaps modify our hypothesis or change the way we approached the hypothesis and try again. It is this iterative process of hypothesis testing, data collection and evaluation that allows science to progress. This is what we are trying to do to understand and prevent suicide. Since its publication in 2011, I and others have tested specific IMV-related hypotheses and some of that research is described in this book.

This brings me to the fifth and final principle that speaks directly to my desire for the model to make a difference in terms of saving lives, by illuminating the pathways from suicidal thoughts to suicidal acts. This principle is probably the most important: although it is all well and good having a theoretical model of suicide, unless it helps us to understand and prevent suicide, it is not worth the paper it is written on. It is this principle that has guided all of the work that I've done since starting out in the mid-nineties. Over the years, I have been humbled when those who have been suicidal or bereaved by suicide have got in touch to tell me that they have found the model helpful, to make sense of their own suicidality or that of their loved ones.

## Suicide as a behaviour

The IMV model was also influenced by the theory of planned behaviour, a theoretical model that is widely used in health psychology.[6] Its inclusion grew out of work that Chris Armitage, a good friend from my PhD days and another health psychologist from the University of Manchester, and I did a few years ago. It builds upon my belief that suicide is best understood as a behaviour and not simply as a by-product of mental illness. In a small study in 2006, we demonstrated that the theory of planned behaviour is a really helpful framework to understand suicidal behaviour.[7]

In brief, the theory of planned behaviour is a social-cognitive psychological model that argues that the immediate predictor of any behaviour is having the intention or motivation to engage in that behaviour. Simply put, if you form an intention to exercise then you are more likely to actually do exercise. An intention, in turn, is predicted by three further psychological factors:

1. Attitudes: these are your beliefs, the extent to which you think positively or negatively about something (e.g., 'I think exercise is a good thing to do').
2. Norms: these are also beliefs, but, this time, they are beliefs about what you believe others think about that behaviour or what you think others do. Keeping with the exercise example, exercise norms tap into whether you believe your family, friends and society think exercise is a good idea.
3. Control: it stands to reason that the more control you think you have over a behaviour the more likely it is that you'll engage in it. Our perceptions of control can be internal ('I believe I have the skills to do the exercise') or external ('I have

the relevant equipment or kit required to engage in exercise'). Internal control is often called self-efficacy and taps into how confident you feel about being able to carry out the behaviour: 'Do I believe I have the capacity to execute the requisite behaviour or behaviours?'

The theory of planned behaviour is thought to be pretty universal and applicable to all behaviours, so we applied it to suicide. We reasoned that in order to attempt suicide, one has to form an intention to engage in suicidal behaviour. This rang true as we knew from a plethora of scientific studies that suicidal intent is a precursor to suicide. Then, in terms of the other three factors, we found in our study that people's attitudes towards suicidal behaviour, the attitudes of their peers and friends towards suicidal behaviour and their self-efficacy (internal control) were associated with suicide risk.[8] Self-efficacy seemed to be particularly strongly associated with future suicidal behaviour. Although ours was only a small study, it demonstrated clearly that these so-called social-cognitive factors are associated with suicide risk and highlights once again that we need to look beyond mental illness to understand suicide risk.

## Risks and Vulnerabilities: The Pre-Motivational Phase

Before moving on to what triggers suicidal ideation, we need to understand the context in which suicidal ideation and behaviour emerge. This brings me back to the pre-motivational phase – phase one of the IMV model. I clearly like triads, as the pre-motivational phase also comprises three components: diathesis (vulnerability), environment and life events.

## Diathesis or vulnerability factors

For the present purposes, diathesis simply means vulnerability. Diathesis is often used to describe a genetic or biological predisposition or vulnerability for a disease, but, in psychology, diathesis is used much more widely; to capture different types of vulnerabilities, including personality and cognitive vulnerabilities. In this section, I touch on biological vulnerability but most of it is dedicated to perfectionism, a personality vulnerability factor that is implicated in suicide risk.[9]

### The role of serotonin

The impairment in regulation of a neurotransmitter (chemical messenger in the brain) such as serotonin would be an example of a biological diathesis or vulnerability factor for suicide. Although changes in serotonin and its metabolites (small molecules) are associated with both depression and suicidal behaviour, serotonin appears to play a distinct role in suicidal behaviour.[10] This is not that surprising given that its effects permeate all facets of our mind and body. It helps us to feel calmer, happier and less anxious, and it is thought to act as a natural mood stabiliser. Therefore, if we have low levels of serotonin circulating in our body, it stands to reason that our mood may be adversely affected.

A group of antidepressant drugs called selective serotonin reuptake inhibitors (SSRIs), which include Prozac and Seroxat, are widely prescribed to tackle this imbalance. They aim to block the reabsorption of serotonin, so that more circulates in the brain, with the aim of combatting low mood. Despite their extensive use, there is debate about the extent to which SSRIs and other pharmacological interventions actually prevent suicide. Overall, the evidence is mixed, with reported anti-suicide effects varying as a function of the type of drug, as well as the age and clinical characteristics of the patient.[11] Often where a drug has been shown to work it is not certain whether the drug is superior to psychological treatment or whether combination treatments are optimal. Moreover, most clinical trials have tended to focus on suicidal ideation and suicide attempts as outcomes rather than suicide. This highlights a wider issue in the field of suicide prevention. As deaths by suicide (thankfully) are statistically rare outcomes, the sample sizes required to establish clinical efficacy are so large that they can be prohibitive. As a consequence, we do not know whether those pharmacological or psychosocial interventions that are not administered en masse actually prevent suicide or not. It is also important to highlight that counter-indications for some drugs have been reported, with possible increases in suicidal ideation evident in some studies, including among those involving patients aged under 25 years.[12] In addition, concerns have been reported by patient advocacy groups, suggesting that the side effects of certain drugs may contribute to suicide risk. For example, akathisia, the movement disorder that renders it difficult to stay still, is a side effect of some antipsychotic medications (these are different from SSRIs) that has been raised as a potential risk factor for suicide. These are legitimate concerns that require closer investigation.

The role of perfectionism

Moving away from biological vulnerabilities, over the past 15 years my team and I have explored the relationship between perfectionism, a personality factor, and suicide risk.[13] Time and again, in one study after another, we have found a particular dimension of perfectionism to be consistently associated with suicidal thoughts and suicide attempts. Indeed, I have been surprised by the robustness of this association. Our programme of research has involved thousands of individuals from different backgrounds and age groups, and has included people from both clinical and community settings. This importance of perfectionism in suicide risk has been supported by a number of reviews over the years.[14] The author Will Storr has also written eloquently about this in the context of male suicide.[15] In a typical study, we assess perfectionism along with other variables including suicidal ideation at one time point – the baseline – and then we go back to these same people at a later date, to investigate the extent to which perfectionism predicts changes in suicidal ideation over time. In our studies as well as those from other research groups, the respondents who rate highly on this particular dimension are more suicidal when we follow them up, usually those who have also experienced high levels of stress during the study period.

The burning question then is, what is this dimension of perfectionism? Before answering, it is worth remembering that, like all personality factors, perfectionism is on a continuum and each of us sits somewhere along this continuum of perfectionistic beliefs. Those who are towards the top end of the continuum are highly perfectionistic and those at the bottom end, less so. It is also worth emphasising that, even among those who score highly, most will be absolutely fine and will never become suicidal. However, it is when life throws up unexpected challenges that perfectionism can start to conspire against us, adversely affecting our mental health.

To answer the question about which type of perfectionism is potentially harmful we need to consider how perfectionism is measured. This tends to be assessed via self-report, with all of the widely used scales assessing multiple dimensions of perfectionism. In our research, we use the Multidimensional Perfectionism Scale developed by Canadian clinical psychologists Paul Hewitt and Gordon Flett.[16] Their scale assesses three different dimensions of perfectionism:

1. Self-oriented perfectionism: the standards we expect of ourselves.
2. Socially prescribed perfectionism: the standards we think others expect of us.
3. Other-oriented perfectionism: our expectations for others to be perfect.

Out of these three dimensions, which do you think is consistently associated with suicide risk? The findings are clear: irrespective of the population studied, high levels of socially prescribed perfectionism (sometimes also referred to as social perfectionism) are reliably associated with suicidal thoughts and suicide attempts across the lifespan. The formal definition of socially prescribed perfectionism involves having unrealistically high expectations of what we believe important people in our lives (significant others) have of us and our behaviour. According to the definition, if we fail to meet such expectations, these people will think badly of us, judging us negatively. People who rate highly on socially prescribed perfectionism tend to believe that those around them expect them to excel in all aspects of life and they (understandably) find it difficult to meet these perceived expectations. In all the studies that I have ever conducted, socially prescribed perfectionism has always been associated with suicide risk.

If we look at the evidence for the other dimensions of perfectionism, the findings are quite muddy. Some studies have found the self-critical aspects of self-oriented perfectionism to be associated with suicide risk, whereas others have suggested that the intrinsic drive characterised by setting high standards for oneself may be protective. It is difficult to judge the role of other-oriented perfectionism as it has been less frequently investigated as a risk factor for suicide. My take on the perfectionism and suicide risk research evidence as a whole is that the findings for self-oriented perfectionism are mixed, other-oriented doesn't seem to play a role, and the suicide risk appears to be largely confined to the socially prescribed perfectionism dimension.

To get a better idea about what we mean by socially prescribed perfectionism, consider the following two items taken from the Multidimensional Perfectionism Scale:

1. 'I find it difficult to meet others' expectations of me.'
2. 'People expect more from me than I am capable of giving.'

We normally ask people to rate the extent to which they agree or disagree with statements such as these on a seven-point scale. In the full scale, there are 15 items, so, when added up, the scale yields a wide range of scores. Take a minute to think about how you would respond to these two items. Don't worry, though, we cannot classify you as a social perfectionist from your responses to these two questions! Even when we use the full scale in our research, our focus is not on a single individual's score, it's on a group of respondents' scores. Usually, we are tracking trends in people's answers and seeking to map these trends on to other factors such as suicidal ideation. Most people score somewhere in the middle on perfectionism scales, which isn't that unexpected, as most of us try to please others, to some degree, at least some of the time. As it happens, I score highly on socially prescribed perfectionism, which didn't come as much of a surprise to me. I am overly concerned about what others expect of me and I spend too much of my waking life worried that I've let others down or ruminating about some potential social faux pas that I may or may not have made.

Given its potential role in suicide risk, it is important to explain what socially prescribed perfectionism is and what it is not. Crucially, it does not tap into the beliefs about what others *actually* expect of us; rather it evaluates what *we think* others expect of us. In psychological terms, these evaluative beliefs are called metacognitions, which is a technical term used to describe having thoughts about thoughts or an understanding of our own thought processes. These metacognitions are a key reason why socially perfectionistic beliefs are potentially damaging, because, by their very nature, they can be inaccurate and seemingly outside of our control. They lead us to believe that important people in our lives have unachievable expectations of us and that they will think less of us if we don't meet these expectations. In most cases, if you are socially perfectionistic, the relationships between what you think others expect of you and what they actually think are unrelated. They are not embedded in real life and, therefore, they are difficult to change.

To illustrate the role of socially prescribed perfectionism a little more, there's a simple metaphor that I often use when I am explaining social perfectionism to an audience: those who score highly on socially prescribed perfectionism have *psychological thin skins* and those who report low levels of socially prescribed perfectionism possess *psychological thick skins*. As we navigate everyday life, if we have a psychological thin skin (like me), when we encounter social threats, such as rejection or defeat or loss, we will experience these much more keenly. And, over time, these experiences may contribute to feelings of low mood and emotional distress – and potentially, in some cases, to the emergence of suicidal thoughts. Social perfectionism is like having a chink in your psychological armour. Although not fatal, it is one vulnerability factor such that when the piercing arrows of social defeat or rejection come our way, they are much more likely to get through our defences. They are much more likely to penetrate our psychological skin.

Take Amanda as an example. Amanda really struggles with what she sees as the pressure to be perfect in the eyes of others:

> Even though part of me knows what I am doing is perfectly okay, I just cannot stop myself thinking that I am not good enough and that if only I worked harder, I'd be able to please them. And even when I think I have done well, I know that I will have to try even harder to do as well the next time.

In many ways, Amanda is the archetypal social perfectionist, caught in a vicious cycle of needing social approval, working tirelessly to obtain it, feeling valued by others, then shifting back again to seeking more approval and pursuing it again and again. It's relentless. It feels to her like a never-ending rollercoaster of highs and lows and, every now and then, she needs a 'time out' and steps off the rollercoaster. Sometimes it gets so bad that she has to stop going out, stop seeing her friends, stop putting herself forward to do things at work because she is so petrified of failing, of letting others down. Then, after some respite, she'll feel rejuvenated and will get back on the rollercoaster again. Although she has never attempted suicide, she still feels overwhelmed a lot of the time, thinking that she's a 'waste of space', periodically feeling suicidal and that she'd be better off dead. When I asked her specifically about times when things felt particularly stressful, she struggled to answer, saying that even the smallest of tasks make her feel anxious and uptight. It is like every task, no matter how small or insignificant, is an opportunity to fail, another opportunity to let others down. I, like many people, definitely know first-hand how Amanda feels.

Amanda's description of being affected by even the most straightforward of tasks illustrates one of the ways in which social perfectionism has its effect on our well-being, as we found out in one of our studies on adolescent self-harm.[17] In that study we investigated the extent to which a number of factors, including perfectionism and negative life events, predicted self-harm over a six-month period in fifteen- to sixteen-year-olds. Before we conducted the study, we hypothesised that the young people who experienced the most negative life events during the six months of the research would be most likely to self-harm. And this is precisely what we found. More surprising, however, was the relationship between socially prescribed perfectionism and risk of self-harm. Whereas we thought that risk of self-harm would be highest among the adolescents who scored high on social perfectionism and also experienced high levels of negative life events, a different pattern of findings emerged. We found that risk of self-harm was elevated among those who reported high levels of perfectionism (not a surprise) and *low levels* of negative life events (a surprise). It is as if a consequence of having high levels of social perfectionism is that the threshold beyond which stressful events become distressing is lowered, which I call the 'stress-threshold lowering effect'. Or it may be easier to think about it in terms of two people who encounter the same stressor: the one with higher levels of perfectionism (the thinner skin) will be more affected by it. These findings were instrumental to my beginning to think about socially prescribed perfectionism in terms of it conferring a metaphorical psychological thin skin on those who score towards the upper end of the scale.

### The role of implicit attitudes

Thus far I have focused on what psychologists call reflective processes and how they can help us to understand suicide risk. However, according to what is called the dual process model, if we are to understand any behaviour, we need to think about two interacting systems. Daniel Kahneman, who won the Nobel Prize for economics, describes these systems brilliantly in his book *Thinking, Fast and Slow*.[18] The first system operates automatically. It is fast, it acts quickly, involving automatic processes and behaviours. The second is the reflective system, which has been the focus of most suicide research. It involves conscious awareness and processing of information. It is slow and effortful, and it reflects our values and attitudes. For example, someone may be deterred from engaging in suicidal behaviour because they think it is morally wrong to end one's life. Or if we think about how trapped we feel, this requires us to *reflect* on a whole range of factors. These are deliberative processes.

The automatic system is not deliberative; it is characterised by habits, impulses and implicit attitudes. The latter are evaluations of ourselves or particular behaviours that occur without conscious awareness. They are distinct from explicit attitudes, which are the attitudes that we are consciously aware of and which we can easily report. So, if I asked you what your (explicit) attitude towards smoking is, you could answer this without much trouble. However, it is much more difficult to tap into implicit beliefs about a particular topic, because we are not consciously aware of them. Or we may not want to disclose our true attitude because others may not approve. For this reason, psychologists have developed innovative experimental techniques to probe these automatic processes. One of the most widely used is the implicit attitudes test (IAT), which taps into our thoughts and feelings that are outside conscious awareness or control.[19] Traditionally, the IAT records the strength of association between concepts (e.g., Irish people) and characteristics (e.g., friendly) using a reaction time task on a computer. The IAT has been used widely to understand racism and sexism, but it wasn't until the past 10–15 years that it was considered for use in understanding suicide risk.

Matt Nock, a clinical psychologist at Harvard University, has led the way in understanding how these automatic processes may be associated with suicide. In 2010, he published a seminal study in which he showed that people seeking treatment at a psychiatric emergency department who had stronger implicit attitudes associating death/suicide with themselves were more likely to attempt suicide in the next six months compared to those with weak associations.[20] What is more, these implicit attitudes were better predictors than well-known risk factors such as depression, and patient and clinician prediction.

A couple of years after this paper was published, I spent some time at Matt's lab in Harvard and this resulted in a joint study led by Christine Cha conducted simultaneously in Scotland and the US.[21] We explored whether it was possible to activate these automatic attitudes towards living or dying in people who had previously thought of suicide. By activate I mean, if we induced low mood in those who took part, would these automatic associations with death versus life get stronger or weaker?

To our mind, this study was important because it helped us to understand whether these automatic processes, such as attitudes towards living or dying, got worse when people felt low or depressed. If so, it could help to uncover why suicide risk escalates and, crucially, it could provide targets for intervention. We used a well-established technique to briefly induce low mood, which involves listening to sad music while reading negative statements. This negative mood induction is completely safe and only makes people feel sad for about 10–20 minutes and, before they leave the lab, we do a positive mood induction and check-in with them to ensure they're feeling okay.

Compared to people who have never been suicidal, we found that those who had been previously suicidal had a weaker identification with living and this association was further weakened after the negative mood induction. What is more, the post-induction IAT scores predicted suicidal thoughts six months later.

Taken as a whole, these findings provide a vital part of the puzzle to understanding suicidal risk. Of course it is important that we ask people how they feel and hear their story, but a focus on these automatic processes gives us further insight into how suicidal thoughts may emerge. They may also be useful if someone is uncertain about how they feel or is reluctant to disclose their suicidal thoughts. But, like all new developments, the ethical issues around tapping into unconscious processes need further exploration.

## The environment and negative life events

We are all products of our environment, therefore, as outlined in the IMV model, if we are to understand suicide risk we need to understand the role of environment in that risk. The field of suicide research and prevention has a long history of trying to characterise those aspects of our environment that are associated with suicide. Environmental influences can take many different forms, ranging from the foetal environment in the womb, through to the familial environment and the wider effects of the community environment, including structural disadvantage, racism and socioeconomic background.[22] However, I want to focus here on the early life environment, in particular upon early life adversity and attachment. Needless to say, adversity occurs across the lifespan, with negative life events in adulthood being associated with suicide risk as well as those experienced during childhood and adolescence.[23]

### Early life adversity

Without doubt, there is a robust relationship between the experience of early life adversity and poor mental health, including suicide risk.[24] Early life adversity can be assessed in many different ways, but it is frequently recorded in terms of adverse childhood experiences (ACEs) that pertain to the first 18 years of life. These experiences include emotional abuse, physical abuse, sexual abuse, exposure to violence directed at a parent, exposure to household substance abuse or household mental illness, parental separation/divorce or having a household member in prison.[25] Numerous studies have shown that as the number of ACEs increases, an individual's health outcomes across the lifespan deteriorate.

In a widely cited American study by Shanta Dube and colleagues, there was a two- to five-fold increase in risk of a suicide attempt for any ACE. More worrying, though, when the ACEs were scored and summed together, a score of 7 or more ACEs increased the likelihood of a suicide attempt in childhood or adolescence by 51-fold and an attempt in adulthood by 30-fold.[26] These are pretty alarming numbers and they are even more concerning when we consider that the relationship between ACEs and suicide attempts still holds after self-reported alcoholism, depression and illicit drug use are statistically accounted for in the analyses.

Another way to think about risk is to quantify the contribution of a risk factor to people getting a disease or, in this case, to attempting suicide. This contribution is known as the population attributable fraction (PAF), or the percentage reduction in suicide attempts that one would expect to see if the risk factor was eliminated from the population. As suicide attempts have multiple and overlapping risk factors, it is not possible to simply add up all of the PAFs to work out how to eliminate suicidal behaviour. Nonetheless, they are a useful tool to guide suicide prevention efforts. In Dube's study, between 80 per cent of childhood or adolescent suicide attempts and 67 per cent of suicide attempts occurring across the lifespan could be attributed to the experience of one or more ACEs. This is high. And although other studies have published different statistics, they all paint the same picture of increasing vulnerability, the greater the exposure to early life trauma. However, the relationship is complex, such that it is still not clear which factors or mechanisms explain the association between childhood adversity and suicide risk.

### The body's response to stress

In terms of biological mechanisms, there is some evidence that these early experiences may alter the expression of genes that, in turn, contribute to vulnerability to mental health problems, thereby increasing the subsequent risk of suicide.[27] Early life adversity may also affect how the body responds to stress via dysregulation of the hypothalamic-pituitary-adrenal (HPA) axis.[28] The HPA axis is central to our body's stress response system; we need it to work well when we encounter stressful situations (otherwise known as stressors). You may have heard of the 'fight or flight response'; this is our body's physiological response to a potential threat or stressor. It is so named because it prepares the body to either fight the threat or flee the situation, as required.

The HPA axis also governs the release of the hormone cortisol, which is known as one of the 'fight or flight' hormones because it is required when we encounter stress. Its release in response to stress is called cortisol stress reactivity. Cortisol has wide-ranging effects on the mind and body that prepare us to combat any threats and it may also be involved in emotion regulation and decision-making. If low levels of cortisol are released in response to stress, this blunted response is thought to be associated with impairment in some aspects of executive function. Executive function is a neuropsychological term to describe a set of mental skills such as working memory, flexible thinking, problem-solving and self-control, each of which helps us to self-regulate. We use these skills all the time as we navigate everyday life, to manage our emotions and to get things done. With regard to suicide risk, if the HPA axis is disrupted, such that not enough cortisol is released, then the body and mind may not be optimally prepared to fight any threats or stressors. The knock-on effect is that the next time we encounter a stressor our response may be less effective, making us more distressed and, over time, potentially making us more vulnerable to suicide.

We have investigated the role of cortisol reactivity in some of our research, with a specific focus on whether people who attempt suicide exhibit a blunted response when under stress compared to those who have only ever thought about suicide or who have never been suicidal at all.[29] This research has been led by my identical twin brother, Daryl O'Connor, who is also a health psychologist and, conveniently for me, an expert in stress research. As a personal aside, I am extremely fortunate to have a twin brother also working as a professor of psychology. Indeed, we have had many fruitful research collaborations since our PhD days; most recently, we reflected on how being identical twins has influenced our professional lives in an interview in The Psychologist.[30]

Getting back to the research. To tap into the cortisol system, we use an experimental procedure to elicit the stress response. There are different ways to do this, but we use a procedure called the Maastricht Acute Stress Test (MAST).[31] This is physiologically as well as psychologically challenging as participants are asked to put their hand in icy cold water and, at the same time, perform a tricky mental arithmetic task in the lab. I know the components of the MAST may sound a bit odd, but these stressors, in combination, are known to activate the HPA axis, therefore they are a good method of investigating how well the stress system is working. We tested this in one of our recent studies by recruiting three groups of people: those who had attempted suicide; those who had thought about suicide; and those who had never been suicidal.[32] Everyone was brought into our lab and, as well as completing some questionnaires, we asked them all to provide samples of saliva before, during and after completing the MAST. In this way, we were able to track the amount of cortisol that they released during the study including while monitoring the effect of the MAST. Precisely as we had predicted, those who had attempted suicide released the lowest amount of cortisol across the study, with those with no suicidal history releasing the greatest amount and those in the suicidal thoughts group sitting somewhere in the middle. In the laboratory setting, therefore, those who had attempted suicide, especially in the past year, exhibited a blunted response when we experimentally induced a stressful situation in the lab. Although I know this experiment is far removed from real life, it gives us some insight into how the stress system will respond in other everyday stressful situations, such as to relationship-or work-related stressors. As well as being psychologically trapped, it seems as though suicidal individuals are also physiologically affected. Unfortunately, we still do not know whether the blunted cortisol response is a cause or consequence of being suicidal; this is another question that needs to be answered.

At the start of this section I suggested that early life adversity may increase suicide risk by affecting the stress response system. So, as a follow-up to the previous study with Daryl, we investigated the extent to which childhood trauma might explain the HPA axis dysregulation in these very same suicidal individuals.[33] When we originally met them in the lab, they had also answered questions about their experience of abuse or neglect in childhood or adolescence and we were able to link their answers to their cortisol data. The findings were clear: those who reported the most childhood trauma released the least amount of cortisol, suggesting their stress reactivity was the most blunted.

Let's take a second to reflect on these findings.

In our study, we asked people to tell us about any abuse or neglect that they may have experienced decades before, and those who self-reported more of these experiences released *less* cortisol in our lab today. Even more shocking is that trauma is really common among those who have attempted suicide. In our sample and in subsequent studies, about 80 per cent of people reported at least one type of childhood trauma.[34] It is also worth remembering that the harmful effects of a blunted cortisol response extend well beyond suicide risk; the former is associated with a wide range of adverse behavioural and health outcomes. We need to do so much more to understand how and why this happens, and what can be done to protect those who are vulnerable.

## Attachment

Although there are biological pathways linking early life trauma to suicide risk, another important pathway to consider is the process of attachment. Attachment relationships are emotional bonds between people that develop early in life and influence relationships throughout adolescence and into adulthood. It is not surprising that disruptions early on in life have the potential to affect these bonds because they act as models for future relationships as we get older. There are different patterns of attachment, with some being adaptive or secure and others being maladaptive or insecure. In the psychological literature, secure attachment, avoidant attachment and anxious attachment (I'll define each in turn shortly) are the most frequently reported attachment styles potentially associated with increased or decreased suicide risk. Avoidant and anxious attachment orientations are often bundled together to describe insecure or maladaptive attachments.

A couple of years ago, I was involved in a review, led by my colleague Tiago Zortea, which examined the extent to which each of these attachment styles was associated with suicide risk.[35] We found 50+ studies and were encouraged to find that in more than 30 of these, higher levels of secure attachment were associated with lower levels of suicidal thoughts or attempts. Good news. So-called secure attachments are thought to be protective because securely attached individuals tend to perceive themselves as being lovable and expect those around them to be caring and responsive to their needs. This is a positive orientation because, more often than not, such individuals feel that their emotional needs are met. Conversely, an individual who has an avoidant orientation tries to maintain distance or autonomy in relationships, as they have a negative view of themselves as well as those around them. Unsurprisingly therefore, such an orientation doesn't often yield nurturing and fulfilling relationships. Sadly, there was clear evidence of avoidant attachments being associated with suicidal thoughts and attempts, and similarly there was a clear relationship found between anxious attachment and suicide risk. An anxious attachment orientation is problematic because the individual is striving for acceptance, but they struggle with receiving affection because they don't think they are worthy or lovable. This type of attachment is also sometimes called preoccupied or ambivalent attachment. Thinking back to socially prescribed perfectionism, it is possible that this type of attachment contributes to a vicious cycle of seeking social approval, not feeling worthy and trying harder and harder to achieve the potentially unattainable. I would have liked to ask Amanda (who seemed to be an archetypal social perfectionist) about her attachment relationships, but I've a good hunch about how she may have responded. In the conclusion of our review, we called for more support focused on attachment-related coping strategies to mitigate against suicide risk.

As part of this programme of research, Tiago also conducted detailed interviews with people who had attempted suicide in the past. The aim of the interviews was to get first-hand experiences of the nature of the relationship between disrupted attachments and suicidal thoughts and behaviours.[36] One of the interviewees, Joanne, aged 22, who had attempted suicide the previous year, gave a powerful account of some of her interpersonal challenges. In this part of the interview, she talks about her early relationships and how they still affect her today:

> I don't trust anyone because I know that people are going to leave. Like my mum left me in the middle of a road, in a car, so she's done that, and she's apparently meant to love me, then what are other people going to do? [ . . .] it's just easier not connecting with someone and just sticking by yourself. If somebody ran me over tomorrow, I'd be pretty ready to go, like, I wouldn't fight it. I'm completely done because everyone's just leaving. There's got to be something wrong with me and I don't know what it is, that's the thing because everyone says that it's not me, but the common factor in everything that's happened is me.

Joanne's sense of abandonment and worthlessness is palpable. She appears to have given up her fight for life and sees suicide as the solution to her interpersonal problems. It is heartbreaking to think that she sees herself as the problem and doesn't seem to be fearful about dying, as if she's resigned to death.

Christina, who was 23, was also interviewed for our study. She had attempted suicide quite a while ago, but she was still taking medication for depression. It was clear that her early life experiences contributed to her sense of entrapment, as she describes below:

> My parents were, like, very abusive to one another and also to me, and that pushed me out of the home, like, from quite an early age anyways. So I was, like, getting into bad stuff, like getting into drugs at the age of 13, and with that came other unpleasant things. So yeah, I felt like I was in this circle, I just felt a bit trapped by life . . . not liking being inside my own brain even, so it's not even like I had a safe space inside myself. It was, kind of, like, I didn't really like myself either, because I didn't like being, yeah, trapped in my brain type thing, I wanted to shut that off.

Christina's descriptions of internal – 'trapped in my brain' – and external– 'a bit trapped by life' – entrapment are poignant and all too common in people who have experienced adversity early on in life. She describes being caught in a cycle of despair, from which there is no respite, and she just cannot find anywhere safe to hunker down to feel safe or to recharge. Similarly, her display of self-dislike, of despondency, is also characteristic of people with insecure attachments and adds to their sense of worthlessness and perception that no one would care if they lived or died.

This lack of self-worth, feeling insignificant and worthless is also mirrored in another transcript, from Matt's interview when he reflects on being suicidal. He's 27 and has attempted suicide twice:

> I had no friends, I had no family and, you know, I'd weighed up all the consequences and the paths and I really couldn't see me living or dying making any impact. I was so depressed at the time and so hopeless at the time [ . . .] then I might as well just go and turn off the lights because it would be easier for me and it's not like I'd be leaving much behind.

At the time of his suicide attempts, he doesn't seem to have any validating relationships in his life and, as a consequence, he has been thinking about the pros and cons of staying alive. His comments are interesting, though, as he recognises that his thoughts about the future ('so hopeless at the time') were blinkered when he 'was so depressed at the time'. This is a powerful reminder that suicidal entrapment is temporary and that things can get better. The challenge, though, is that in the depths of despair, it is difficult to see that. Matt's initial comment about having no friends or family also brings to mind John Donne, the seventeenth-century Jacobean poet's quote that 'No man is an island, entire of itself'. It highlights the vital importance of human connection and that, when connectedness is thwarted, then suicide risk is increased.[37]

## Suicidal Thoughts and the Motivational Phase

If you are supporting someone who is struggling, the IMV model should help you to identify warning signs that they may be feeling suicidal or at risk of suicide. Specifically, it helps us to distinguish between people who feel suicidal but are less likely to attempt suicide and those who are at greater risk of taking the next step and engaging in a suicidal act. Clearly this distinction is of paramount importance, as it is critical that we better understand who is most vulnerable, and who is most likely to attempt suicide or ultimately die by suicide. This transition is captured by the motivational and volitional phases, which deal with suicidal ideation and suicide attempts, respectively. As I've outlined already, the factors in the motivational phase drive the emergence of suicidal ideation. Specifically, suicidal ideation results from feelings of defeat and/or humiliation from which you cannot escape. If you take a look at Figure 1 again (page 102), just below defeat, entrapment and suicidal ideation you'll see boxes entitled 'threat to self moderators', 'motivational moderators' and 'volitional moderators'. These contain the key factors that help us to understand how someone moves from feeling defeated and humiliated to ultimately engaging in suicidal behaviour.

A moderator is a statistical term used to describe a factor that may affect the direction and/or strength of the relationship between two other factors. Thinking about the relationship between stress and well-being is a good place to start to illustrate what I mean by a moderator. Imagine if someone you know feels stressed and they have no one to turn to for support, then the likelihood that they will become distressed is higher than if they had someone to turn to. This is because having someone to turn to, having social support, is a good thing. It may help them to cope with the stress they are experiencing, thereby reducing the likelihood that they become distressed. In this example, having social support is acting as a moderator, as it changes (reduces) the likelihood that stress leads to distress.

If you look again at Figure 1 (see page 102), below the moderators are three further boxes that list a range of psychological factors, each feeding into one of the moderator boxes above. Take the 'threat to self moderators', for example – they comprise psychological processes like social problem-solving, coping and memory biases. The presence of each of these moderators or factors is hypothesised to affect the relationship between defeat/humiliation and entrapment so that their presence, if negative, will make it more likely that an individual feels trapped by their feelings of defeat or humiliation. In such cases, an individual moves figuratively from left to right in the model and, in so doing, their likelihood of suicidal ideation and behaviour increases. Also, when we are feeling low in mood, the way we remember things from our past can become distorted so that we are more likely to remember negative rather than positive things. This is problematic because this can exacerbate feelings of entrapment as our mind becomes clogged up with aversive memories. These distortions, called autobiographical memory biases, can also interfere with our capacity to solve social problems.[38] This can happen because we often rely on specific details when we solved a particular social problem from the past to help us solve a new problem now. But when we are low in mood or suicidal, the bias unhelpfully stops us from remembering the relevant details, which results in us being less effective problem-solvers and more likely to feel trapped.[39]

Let's consider Isaac, 32, who is single and lives alone. His story is a good example of how memory biases can affect problem-solving. He has been in regular contact with his GP because he feels really low and suicidal, which he blames, in part, on a family rift. Other experiences from his past, including workplace bullying, have also contributed to his low mood. As a consequence of the rift, he is estranged from his mother and father and, although he really wants to foster reconciliation, he just cannot work out how to make this happen. There have been previous family rifts that have been successfully resolved, but when I ask him, he struggles to recall the specific details of how these were achieved. However, he can talk in great detail about negative things related to his family circumstances. In terms of the autobiographical memory biases, therefore, Isaac's story is typical. He is more likely to remember negative rather than positive memories and, to make matters worse, his positive memories of the previous reconciliations are over-general; they lack the detail required to help him to think about strategies to problem-solve his current family crisis.

## Disrupting pathways to entrapment and suicidal thoughts

Let's try to unpack the motivational phase a little more by thinking about a time in your life when you initially felt defeated by a social (interpersonal) situation. Pick one that you were able to resolve, that ended positively. It could have been a problem at work or at school or an incident with friends:

- What was it?
- What did you do to solve the problem?

Take a few minutes to think about such a situation.

It may also be helpful to consider a hypothetical scenario and relate it back to the IMV model:

> Imagine you are repeatedly clashing with a work colleague, resulting in you feeling that your voice is never heard. These clashes become more and more heated to such an extent that you don't know how to resolve the situation and all of your energy is consumed by managing your emotions after each encounter. These clashes are really getting you down, you are feeling pretty defeated and trapped by the situation as every meeting ends in a heated argument. You are stuck in a rut, not knowing what to do. However, after speaking with a friend, you are encouraged to broach the issue with your colleague in an open and non-judgemental way. Raising the issue is helpful as you discover that you remind your colleague of a previous co-worker who had been quite abusive. As a result, your colleague always feels uptight in your presence, which manifests itself as argumentative behaviour. However, by naming the issue you are able to resolve it together.

Now let's dissect this scenario in terms of the IMV model.

First, by resolving the recurrent arguments, the pathway (or link) from defeat to entrapment became less likely. Being able to resolve the problem *moderated* the relationship between defeat and entrapment so that the solution made it less likely that you continued to feel trapped. In general, moderators can act in two ways: they can weaken a relationship or they can strengthen it. In the example above, effective problem-solving, which psychologists may also describe as problem-focused coping, weakened the relationship between defeat and entrapment.

Conversely, if you had responded differently to the situation, perhaps by just digging your heels in without trying to resolve the issue, then such a response may have made it more likely that you'd continue to feel trapped, thereby strengthening the defeat to entrapment pathway. Both weakening and strengthening are examples of moderation. When a moderator is protective, we often describe it as a buffer. We all need buffers in our lives!

Why not try to frame the situation you thought about earlier (the problem at work or school or with friends), when you felt defeated, in terms of the factors within the IMV model? Did you use any of the threat to self moderators to resolve your defeating situation? How did you cope with any distress you experienced?

Now let's move on to the entrapment to suicidal ideation pathway. Whereas 'threat to self moderators' are focused on the transition from defeat to entrapment, the 'motivational moderators' are the group of factors that increase or decrease the likelihood that feelings of entrapment lead to suicidal ideation. For example, thwarted belongingness, feeling a burden on others, having few positive thoughts for the future and having little social support render it more likely that suicidal ideation will emerge out of the despair of entrapment. But it is important to note that suicidal ideation is not an inevitable consequence of entrapment and that not all motivational moderators make matters worse. Some are protective; as noted above, they're buffers. Most people who experience entrapment will not become acutely suicidal. Crucially, if we are able to intervene to target those factors that do us harm, we can protect those who feel trapped. The challenge, though, is spotting who is feeling trapped and knowing how and when to intervene to keep them safe. I'll return to how we can help to keep people safe in Part 3.

## The role of positive thoughts about the future

Perhaps unsurprisingly, our thoughts about the future are also important to help us navigate through the darkness, when hopelessness descends. If we are feeling trapped, for example, suicidal thoughts are more likely to emerge if we have nothing positive to look forward to. For this reason, future thoughts are included as a motivational moderator within the IMV model. Building upon the work of Andrew MacLeod, we have spent many years trying to unpick the nature of the relationship between future thinking and suicide risk. MacLeod, a clinical psychologist at Royal Holloway, University of London, pioneered this work in the nineties. Specifically, he developed the 'future thinking task', which is a relatively straightforward verbal task that involves people naming the things that they are looking forward to or worried about in the future.[40] This task allows us to tap into people's positive and negative future thoughts, respectively. Positive thoughts can include anything from 'going on holiday' to 'seeing my boyfriend' or 'going out for dinner'. Whereas negative thoughts such as 'having an argument with my partner', 'losing my job' or 'becoming ill' are typical of the answers people give for what they're worried about.

MacLeod's initial findings were striking. When he asked people who had self-harmed or attempted suicide about their future thoughts and compared their answers to others who were not suicidal, a clear pattern emerged. Suicidal individuals had fewer positive future thoughts compared to those who had never been suicidal and they also had fewer positive thoughts relative to people who were depressed. Moreover, there didn't seem to be any differences in their negative future thinking. We, and other research groups, have also found this absence of positive future thinking in those who attempt suicide.[41] More recently, we have shown that the degree to which people can think of positive future events predicts recovery in the weeks following a suicide attempt – those who can only think of a few positive future thoughts immediately after a suicide attempt are much more suicidal two months later compared to those who can think of more positive future thoughts.[42] So, positive future thoughts tend to be protective in the short term.

Like most things in life, the relationship between positive future thoughts and suicidal behaviour is more complicated than we had originally thought, however. The long-story-short is that, whereas positive future thoughts seem to be protective in the weeks following a suicide attempt, particular types of thoughts may counter-intuitively contribute to one's darkness in the medium term if those positive future thoughts are not attainable. This is the conclusion I came to after one of our studies in which we tracked people for up to 15 months following a suicide attempt.[43] In brief, we found that those who have high levels of what we call 'intrapersonal' positive future thoughts were more likely to attempt suicide again. Intrapersonal future thoughts are thoughts that only involve the individual and not others and include things such as 'I want to be recovered', 'I want to be more confident' or 'I want to be happy'. For example, our concern is that if, over time, one of the person's positive future thoughts is 'recovery from depression' and then they don't recover, this failure may contribute to feelings of entrapment. Then they're back into the entrapment–suicidal thoughts–entrapment cycle of despair.

When we are trying to understand suicide risk, I think there are two key conclusions here. First, in general, having positive thoughts for the future is a good thing and we should help people as much as possible to think about hopes and aspirations for the future. Second, when considering positive future thoughts it is important to be realistic, so that if specific hopes or positive future thoughts are not achievable, it may be worth thinking about different future aspirations. We need to be more self-accepting and self-compassionate of our own shortcomings and remind ourselves that everyone experiences failure, which is okay and is part of the wider human condition. Indeed, my Glasgow colleague Seonaid Cleare led a review of the research literature on the relationship between self-compassion and suicidal ideation.[44] Although we only found a few studies, the findings were clear: self-compassion and self-forgiveness are protective.

### Applying the motivational phase to understanding people's lives

To end this section, here are two stories that illustrate the harmful and protective effects, respectively, of some motivational moderators:

Charlotte, in her thirties, came up to me at the end of a talk I gave. Although she has never attempted suicide, she has lived with suicidal thoughts for many years. She has traced her problems back to feeling like she has never belonged anywhere and has struggled to fit in all of her life; she has always felt like an outsider. She lives in a rural community and is transgender and her parents disowned her when she started to transition. She has a long history of mental health problems, stretching back to her teens. She told me that, although the dysphoria associated with her gender-identification had improved since transitioning, she still felt psychologically trapped. Despite no longer feeling 'trapped within her body', she was still in emotional pain, feeling emotionally imprisoned. She just longed for her parents to accept her as Charlotte. She just wanted to belong, to feel valued, to be treated as a cherished part of her family.

In terms of the IMV model, it was the thwarted desire to belong, in conjunction with feelings of entrapment, that were exacerbating her suicidal thoughts. Thankfully, she was in a pretty good place when I met her, but Charlotte's suicidal thoughts may come and go until her thwarted sense of belonging is resolved. It seems to be this lack of belonging that is damaging and moderating, or reinforcing, the entrapment to suicidal ideation relationship.

Ava, on the other hand, had acted on her thoughts, having attempted suicide once before in her late teens. Now aged 24, she told me that she felt safe, in that she didn't think she was a danger to herself any longer. Again, her story is not uncommon. She was bullied at school, suffered from low self-esteem and, to this day, she finds it difficult to make and keep friends. She harbours a deep sense of guilt though because, in her eyes, she was a 'difficult' teenager. She had a few spells in trouble with the police in her mid-teens and regrets causing her parents so much pain and anguish. A few days before her twentieth birthday, she had had enough. She remembers feeling that she was nothing but a burden on her family, that no one would miss her if she was dead, that everything she did was wrong and she just wanted it all to stop. The next thing she remembers is waking up in hospital, with no idea where she was or how she got there. Fortunately, Ava survived her suicide attempt and was referred to a psychiatric nurse specialist. This was a turning point for her, as she really connected with her nurse, who arranged for her GP to refer her for an autism assessment. When I met her, she said she was doing well, and had a renewed sense of self-worth following her autism diagnosis. She no longer felt that she was a burden on her family.

'Everything makes sense to me now,' she beamed, as she now has a language to understand how she felt and why she has struggled socially for all these years. She had felt that her family thought she was 'strange' and 'unpredictable', but now she didn't feel like that, as she was 'no longer a problem for them'. Everything had changed for her, as she was now at college, taking a course in finance, buoyed up by having a real purpose in life. Crucially, she no longer feels that she is a burden on her family. Despite sometimes still feeling trapped, her distress is manageable and it no longer escalates into thoughts of death. Ava's story illustrates the protective effects of targeting burdensomeness, another motivational moderator, and it illustrates that, for some, the causes of suicidal thoughts can be identified and their effects neutralised.

As an aside, Ava's story reflects a wider issue. Up until recently, there was little recognition that people with autism spectrum conditions are at increased risk of suicidal thoughts and behaviours. Understanding precisely why remains unclear, but recent research by psychologists Sarah Cassidy and Simon Baron-Cohen points to camouflaging – the tendency to mask one's autistic spectrum characteristics to cope with social situations – together with unmet support needs as being uniquely associated with suicidality.[45] It is also recognised that deaths by suicide associated with autism are also likely to be under-reported. Much more work is needed to understand the unique risks as well as what protects autistic individuals against suicide.[46] And we need to do more to help trans young people like Charlotte.[47]

This chapter has focused primarily on the pathways to the emergence of suicidal thoughts. I hope it has helped you to understand how and why suicidal thoughts emerge as well as to identify warning signs that you should look out for in those around you. In the next chapter, I will deal with the volitional phase of the IMV model, which tackles the important topic of why some people act on their thoughts of suicide and others do not.

# Crossing the Precipice: From Thoughts of Suicide to Suicidal Behaviour

I never thought he'd do it. A few weeks before his death, he had told me that he had thoughts about being dead, but I was too scared to ask him directly whether he would kill himself. I haven't stopped asking myself why I didn't ask him. Not a day passes when I don't torment myself with this question. When I look back on it now, I just didn't think he was the type of person who would kill himself. I know how ridiculous that sounds, but he was just always so full of life.

This is part of a conversation that I had with a heartbroken mother about a year after her son's death. It illustrates just how incredibly difficult it is to identify *a priori* who will act on their suicidal thoughts and who will not. As we endeavour to improve our ability to predict suicidal behaviour, we should never stop striving to protect those who are vulnerable. Every one of us who works in suicide research and prevention grapples with this greatest of challenges daily – of identifying, among those who think about suicide, who is more likely to attempt suicide. The volitional phase of the IMV model (see page 142) is my attempt to do so, to make sense of the transition from thinking about suicide to attempting suicide. The term volitional phase is widely used in psychology and it is defined as the phase after an individual has formed their intention to engage in any behaviour. The motivational phase, on the other hand, describes the processes that lead to the formation of one's intention to engage in a behaviour.

This phase of the IMV model seeks to pinpoint the specific factors that mark out the approximately one third of people who traverse the suicidal precipice, making the transition from suicidal thoughts to a suicidal act.[1] When someone acts, it is the potential lethality of the suicide method – the 'case fatality rate' (the number of suicides by that method divided by the number of suicide attempts by the same method) – that will influence whether the act is fatal or not. Chance or serendipity may also play a role in determining whether or not the suicidal act results in death.

In this chapter I will take you through the things to look out for that may suggest someone is thinking about acting on their thoughts of suicide. This includes some of the questions that should help you to probe the likelihood of a suicidal act.

The volitional phase comprises the eight key factors, as shown in Figure 2 below, that are associated with an increased likelihood that someone will act upon their thoughts of suicide. This more detailed description of the volitional phase was added when I updated the model with my colleague and friend Olivia Kirtley in 2018.[2] Immediately below each factor in Figure 2 I have also included a question to help you think about whether this relates to someone you know. These factors are akin to bridges between suicidal ideation and suicidal behaviour. Whereas we normally build bridges to be sturdy and safely span points A to B, in this case, we want to have these metaphorical bridges in our sights, and then do whatever we can to blow these bridges up to ensure that as few people as possible make

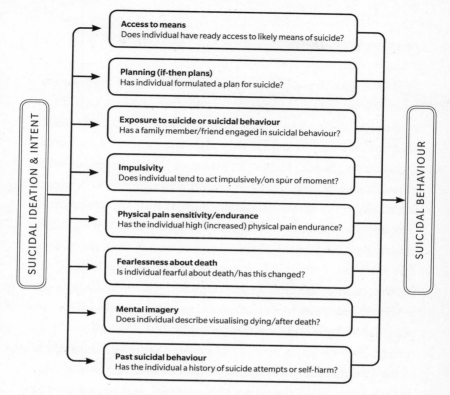

Figure 2. The eight volitional factors: the transition from suicidal ideation to suicidal behaviour[3]

the crossing from suicidal thoughts to suicidal behaviour. As you'll see, these volitional factors can be environmental, social, psychological or physiological in nature.

After a TED-style talk I gave at the American Association of Suicidology Conference in Washington, DC, in 2018, one of the delegates, Ken Norton, described these eight factors as the 'eight hallmarks that bridge suicidal thoughts and actions' on Twitter.[4] I really like this description and have stuck with it ever since as I think it really captures the essence of what I mean by volitional factors. Let's take each hallmark in turn.

## Access to Means

First up is access to the means of suicide. This is an environmental volitional factor. If someone is thinking of ending their life, it is perhaps not surprising that if they have ready access to their preferred method of suicide they are more likely to act on their thoughts of suicide. Indeed, in terms of the evidence for what prevents suicide, the strongest research evidence is for restricting access to the means of suicide.[5] Simply put, any intervention that imposes environmental, social or psychological barriers to enacting a suicidal act will help to save lives. A clear example of this emerged in the UK some years ago from an unexpected source. Before the fifties, the domestic gas used in people's homes was derived from coal and it was toxic, and sadly many people died by suicide via this means of carbon monoxide poisoning. However, with the introduction of non-toxic natural gas in the UK in the late fifties, the number of suicides by such poisoning decreased in the sixties and seventies. Indeed, it has been estimated that between 6,000 and 7,000 lives were saved as a result of this change in gas provision.[6]

The effect of the introduction of natural gas on suicide rates was described in a seminal study led by Edinburgh-based psychiatrist Norman Kreitman, which highlighted that, on the whole, if we restrict access to a particular method of suicide then it does not lead to what is known as a 'substitution effect'.[7] In the case of carbon monoxide, when such deaths decreased there was only a small increase in suicides by other methods. Overall, people tend not to substitute the restricted method for another method of suicide in the short term. However, it is important to be vigilant in case new methods of suicide start to emerge.[8]

There are other public health innovations that have directly or indirectly led to reductions in suicides over the years. These include the installation of catalytic converters on car exhausts, tighter regulations on the import and sale of pesticides, and legislation to restrict the sale of paracetamol and other analgesic tablets to blister packs of 16.[9] In the UK the paracetamol legislation was introduced in 1998 and, some years later, University of Oxford psychiatrist Keith Hawton demonstrated that, after the introduction of this legislation, there was a 43 per cent reduction in such deaths involving paracetamol.[10]

More recently, Jane Pirkis from the University of Melbourne, a good friend with whom I now co-edit *The International Handbook of Suicide Prevention*, and her colleagues explored whether interventions at areas of concern, such as bridges, are effective in preventing suicide. Jane and her colleagues reviewed three types of interventions: those that restrict access to means (e.g., installation of barriers or nets on bridges), those that encourage help-seeking (e.g., installation of signage directing distressed individuals to crisis helplines), and those that increase the likelihood that a third party might intervene to save a life (e.g., installation of CCTV cameras at areas of concern).[11] In their review, they found evidence that each of these interventions was associated with a reduction in deaths from suicide at these sites of concern. Despite these promising findings, however, we still don't know whether such interventions, when rolled out in combination, are more effective than interventions delivered in isolation. It is also not clear whether the various interventions are effective equally across different vulnerable groups. Nonetheless, these are real life-saving interventions targeting the volitional phase and illustrate the potential benefits of such large-scale interventions.

## Planning or If-Then Plans

Next, if a loved one is having thoughts of suicide, top of the list of questions to ask is whether they have formulated a plan for suicide. If the answer is yes, the next question is how specific their plan is and whether they have ready access to the means to enact the plan. If the answers to these questions are yes and the person is saying that they don't know whether they can keep themselves safe, then the time to act is now. If you don't think you can keep the person safe yourself, get in touch with a GP or a mental health professional and, if necessary, contact the emergency services.

Returning to the nuts and bolts of suicide planning, clearly this volitional factor is related to access to means because if they have formulated a specific plan *and* they have access to those specific means, then the likelihood that they'll cross the precipice is increased because the environmental constraints have been reduced or removed. Indeed, we know from extensive psychological research into goal-directed health behaviours that if someone formulates what is called an *implementation* intention (e.g., 'I intend to eat healthily next week by consuming five portions of fruit and vegetables every day') then they are more likely to carry out the behaviour compared to someone who only forms a *goal* intention (e.g., 'I intend to eat healthily').[12] The same applies to suicidal behaviour. Implementation intentions comprise if-then plans because they specify when and where a particular goal-directed behaviour will be enacted. They are called if-then plans because they tap into the triggers for a given behaviour and the associated response to such triggers (e.g., '*IF* I feel stressed *THEN* I eat unhealthy snacks').

They can help us to identify prompts for different behaviours that, in turn, can be translated into better support for those who wish to engage in or avoid specific behaviours.

Often, when we think about implementation intentions in public health terms, we are seeking to encourage health-protective behaviours such as promoting healthy eating or doing exercise. However, in the context of suicide prevention we're trying to do the opposite. We don't want people to engage in suicidal behaviour (the 'then') when they are feeling distressed (the 'if'). We are trying to break the link between the 'if' and the 'then', and usually we are seeking to redraw the 'if-then' linkages, so that suicidal behaviour is less likely to be the response to any of the triggers. To this end, implementation intentions are beneficial to suicide prevention in two regards. First, and obviously, they help us to understand whether an individual has formulated a suicide plan (what is the plan, when and where will it take place) or not – and with this information hopefully we can help to keep more people safe. In Chapter 10 I describe more safety planning techniques to help protect us against suicide.

The second benefit of if-then plans is that they are useful techniques to encourage someone to break the links between existing triggers and subsequent suicidal behaviour. If we think about suicidal acts as behaviours, we know that those who engage in a suicidal act once are statistically more likely to do so again. In other areas of psychology, it is well established that past behaviour is the best predictor of future behaviour. This is, in part, because when we engage in any behaviour, we lay down a memory trace linking the trigger to that behaviour. As a result, the next time we come across that same trigger, it is likely to elicit the same response. If we think about someone whose previous suicide attempt was triggered by feeling trapped by mental pain, if they feel trapped again, then they are at increased risk of engaging in suicidal behaviour again and potentially dying by suicide.

Chris Armitage and I wanted to exploit these if-then linkages to *reduce* suicidal behaviour. Building upon work that Chris had done previously with other health behaviours, in a couple of studies, we embedded if-then plans in a bespoke Volitional Help Sheet (VHS).[13] The VHS is one side of an A4 sheet of paper that lists 12 common triggers or situations when individuals are tempted to engage in suicidal behaviour, ranging from 'I want to get relief from a terrible state of mind' to 'I feel trapped' or 'I feel hopeless'. These are listed in a single column. However, the VHS also lists 12 potential solutions in another adjacent column, and these solutions are derived from clinical psychology and outline therapeutic techniques that have been shown to be helpful in other clinical settings. These solutions are the 'then' responses in the context of 'if-then planning', and they include everything from distraction techniques ('then I will do something else instead') to reaching out for social support ('then I will seek out someone who listens when I need to talk') and taking medication. The function of the help sheet is to encourage individuals to reflect upon the triggers for their suicidal behaviour and then to link these triggers to different responses (i.e., not self-harm) by drawing lines between the situations and the solutions. The participants are also encouraged to make as many or as few situation–solution links as they'd like. By making these linkages the idea is that the next time they feel trapped (situation), their response won't be self-harm or suicidal behaviour, but instead they'll opt for another solution, for example, by seeking out someone who will listen.

We are trying to use the help sheet to facilitate the search for new potential solutions. However, given the complexity of the factors that lead to suicidal behaviour, a single brief help sheet intervention is not going to prevent suicide or self-harm, but it could be a useful tool as an addition to usual care, helping to nudge people away from suicidal behaviour when they are in the midst of a crisis. It is also important to emphasise, therefore, that I am not, for one second, trying to condense the treatment of suicidal behaviour or self-harm into a simple help sheet. Indeed, at the time when Chris and I first discussed tailoring the VHS for use with suicidal individuals I was a little sceptical. However, the VHS approach does seem to help some people to reflect upon their suicidal triggers and consider alternative responses, and, as a result, it does have merit for some people some of the time. Like all potential solutions, though, they are only suitable for certain people. I see the VHS as only one of many tools that could play a small role in reducing the likelihood that someone crosses the suicidal precipice from thoughts to suicidal acts (see Part 3).

In terms of the evidence for the VHS, we have conducted two studies with people treated in hospital following suicidal behaviour, both of which have yielded encouraging findings. One of the studies was conducted in Malaysia.[14] It was exploratory and had some methodological challenges, but its findings pointed to reduced risk of suicidal behaviour among those who completed the VHS. The other study, conducted in Scotland, involved a fully randomised clinical trial (RCT) with patients who had been admitted to hospital following a suicide attempt.[15] When we followed up the participants six months later, we found that the VHS did not seem to have any effect on the total number of people who were subsequently hospitalised for self-harm.

However, when we did some additional analyses, an interesting pattern of findings emerged. We discovered that among those patients who had actually completed the help sheet and who had been previously hospitalised for self-harm before taking part in our study, the VHS appeared to be effective. Although this group of patients didn't stop self-harming completely, the number of times that they self-harmed during the six months of the study period was less than the number for those who only received their usual treatment. These are encouraging findings. However, more research is required to double-check the extent to which the VHS is useful for those with a past history of self-harm.

## Exposure to Suicide or Suicidal Behaviour

As someone who has been bereaved twice by suicide, I have spent considerable time thinking about this third volitional factor and its impact on my own risk of suicide. I have also thought a lot about the impact on my children, not only of being exposed to suicide vicariously through the work that I do, but the effect of the death of my close friend Clare on my children's risk of suicide. My fears and concerns are pretty universal when it comes to suicide bereavement. Indeed, I have yet to meet anyone bereaved by suicide who hasn't been frightened about the potential knock-on transmission of suicide risk to their offspring or those close to them.

When I first met Angela Samata, the presenter of *Life After Suicide*, the BAFTA-nominated documentary and winner of the Mind Media Award for Best Factual TV documentary, this was one of the first questions she asked me, 'Are my children at risk of suicide?'[16] Angela had lost her partner to suicide more than a decade before and, as the mother of two children, one of her biggest fears was that her kids would take their lives, influenced in part by their father's death by suicide. I tried to reassure her by highlighting that suicide is not caused by a single factor and that, although there is a risk, it is important to put this risk in context. *Life After Suicide* is such a powerful film. In it, Angela travels across the UK meeting people who have been bereaved by suicide, exploring the devastating impact of suicide, the stigma they experience and efforts to understand this most complex of phenomena.

I acted as an advisor to the BBC on the film and I was one of the people whom Angela met on her on-screen journey. I talked about the research that we have done to understand why people die by suicide. Although my main contribution was professional, during the course of filming, Leo Burley, the director, asked whether I would share my own experience of suicide bereavement on camera. I was initially reluctant as I had never shared these personal experiences in a public forum before, but after some consideration I agreed and I am so pleased that I did. The feedback I received about my own personal disclosure was heart-warming and it seemed to help others.[17] From that day on, I resolved to be open about my own losses and their impact on me, both personally as well as professionally. Actually, I don't think I would have written this book if I hadn't talked about my own experience of bereavement in the film. The reach of such programmes is vast; *Life After Suicide* was first broadcast in 2015 and it has since been viewed by over 5 million people worldwide. Another great example is *Man Up*, a documentary series and campaign funded by the charity Movember and broadcast in Australia in 2016. It was viewed by 2.6 million Australians, and Jane Pirkis and her colleagues in Melbourne were able to show in a study launched to coincide with its broadcast that the documentary increased the likelihood that men would reach out for help if they were struggling.[18]

When Angela asked me about the risk to her children – and to others including herself – of losing a close loved one to suicide, I started by emphasising that the relationship between exposure and suicide is complicated. Without question, there is evidence that having someone close to you die by suicide is associated with an increased risk of dying by suicide yourself.[19] In a review of the research evidence published in 2014, Alexandra Pitman and colleagues from University College London concluded that there is an increased risk of suicide in partners bereaved by suicide and in mothers bereaved by an adult child.[20] They also noted that there is an increased risk of depression in offspring bereaved by the suicide of a parent. There is also good evidence that parental suicide is associated with offspring suicide, with risk greater after maternal than paternal suicide, and if the death happens when the offspring is at a younger age.[21] Moreover, in another more recent review published in 2020, the association between parental suicide and suicidal behaviour in adult offspring was further reinforced.[22]

It is important to note, however, that exposure itself does not cause suicide. Its effect is more indirect and, as I've said several times, suicide is never caused by a single factor. In terms of the IMV model, exposure acts as a social volitional factor that increases the likelihood someone will act on their thoughts of suicide. Beyond the understandable effects of bereavement, exposure does not directly make someone suicidal per se. Clearly, if a parent takes their life, the experience is traumatic, especially as a child. The same holds for the loss of a partner. In addition to the trauma and the pain of bereavement, there are specific mechanisms that explain how exposure may increase risk. It may increase risk via the process of social modelling. Being exposed to the suicidal behaviour of someone close to us, or to someone with whom we identify (e.g., someone who is the same age or has the same background), increases the likelihood that we may imitate or model that same behaviour. This so-called social modelling is as true for suicidal behaviour as it is for any other behaviour. For each of us, our own behaviour is influenced by the behaviour of others.

Psychologists and other researchers also talk about cognitive accessibility or cognitive availability as another potential mechanism linking exposure to suicide risk.[23] If a close friend or family member attempts or dies by suicide, then naturally we spend time thinking about and talking about suicide, and this gives suicide a cognitive salience that perhaps it didn't have previously. This salience may, in turn, make suicide more cognitively accessible and make it more likely that it will enter our consciousness when times get tough in the future. It is this cognitive accessibility that may, in part, render suicide as a possible solution, as a means of ending one's pain.

Before moving on, I'd like to offer some reassurance: the overwhelming majority of people who are bereaved by or exposed to suicide will never become suicidal and will certainly never end their lives. This reminds me of a family whom I met a few months after the death of their son, who took his own life in his mid-twenties. In the weeks following their son's death, the mother went to see a counsellor and, although her recollection is hazy, she left one of the appointments petrified and in distress because she was told by the counsellor that their other child's risk of suicide had doubled as a result of the bereavement. After exploring this a little with the mother, what I managed to piece together was that the counsellor had misunderstood the difference between relative and absolute risk. These are statistical terms that I'll try to explain. Of course it is frightening to hear that your or a loved one's risk of any disease (e.g., cancer) or adverse outcome (e.g., suicide) has doubled, but what does that actually mean? To make sense of any 'doubling' in risk, let's consider the following example of what absolute risk and relative risk mean. The absolute risk of someone in a population who *has not* been bereaved dying by suicide might be 10 in 100,000, whereas the absolute risk of someone who *has* been bereaved dying by suicide might be 20 in 100,000. If we express this in terms of relative risk of suicide, it does sound incredibly scary, because the risk of suicide in those bereaved seems to be double that of those not bereaved. However, if we go back to the absolute risk figures, the absolute risk or likelihood of suicide is still relatively low. In this hypothetical case, in terms of suicide rates, an absolute risk rate of 20 in 100,000 means that for every 100,000 people in a population, 20 will die by suicide. So although every single death by suicide is a tragedy and the risk is real in statistical terms, it remains small, and mitigating subsequent risk is a real balancing act. It is also important to remember that suicide results from a complex interplay of factors, not just one factor, and risk varies by age, background and relationship with the person who died.[24]

## Social media

Exposure to suicide and self-harm can take many different forms. In recent years, there has been an avalanche of media reports blaming social media use for all of society's ills including suicide and self-harm. Like all things in life, the relationship between social media (Instagram, Facebook, Twitter, TikTok, for example) and well-being is much more complicated than is commonly reported. Without question, excessive social media use is not beneficial and it is potentially dangerous to those who are already vulnerable. And I strongly advocate for social media platforms to be made as safe as possible, to safeguard all of us.

Sadly though, when the tragic suicide deaths of young people are reported, too often the media coverage is misleading. It reduces the myriad causes of suicide to a single factor, too often to social media. Indeed, this is precisely how the increases in child and adolescent suicide risk in the US were presented in the Netflix documentary-drama *The Social Dilemma*.[25] I appreciate that the aim of the programme was to sound alarm bells about the dangers of excessive social networking and this, in itself, is laudable. And I found the programme engaging and informative, in parts. However, I was disappointed by the simplistic, evidence-light way in which a topic as important as youth suicide, which affects so many, was portrayed. The producers presented some really frightening statistics from the Centers for Disease Control and Prevention in the US. They reported that, since 2009, the rates of self-harm have increased by 62 per cent in 15–19-year-old girls and by 189 per cent in 10–14-year-old girls. Even more concerning, they highlighted that compared to the average rates between 2001 and 2010, suicide rates have increased by 70 per cent in girls aged 15–19 years and by 151 per cent in girls aged 10–14 years.[26] These statistics are horrifying and, as I said earlier, there have also been increases in suicides among young females in the UK.

Of course, online bullying or cyber-shaming will be contributory factors in some of these tragic deaths, but there is no evidence that the stark increases can be laid squarely at the door of social media.[27] What is more, as some of the contributors also highlighted in the programme, I am concerned about the extent to which our self-worth and identity are bound up in social approval that is 'dosed to us' on social media. Not to mention the adverse impact that social media use may have on sleeping when heavy use is at night, as sleep is so integral to our mental health. Indeed, earlier I talked about the vicious cycle of the pursuit of social approval and its relationship with socially prescribed perfectionism that I, and many of us, struggle with daily, irrespective of our social media use (see page 126).

In *The Social Dilemma*, however, we were told 'that [the] pattern [of suicides/self-harm] points to social media', but I beg to differ. Notwithstanding the caveat noted above, there is no evidence to support this simplistic assertion. No attempt whatsoever was made to provide the wider social context that may also explain the increase. Although I understand that it can be difficult to present nuance in a docudrama and that screen time is limited, the programme-makers have a responsibility to get the facts right when it relates to such an important public health issue. The short answer is that we do not know for certain why the suicide rates are increasing among young girls and, without doubt, social media will feature, but more likely as an indirect rather than a direct risk factor. What we do know, however, is that the years of increase coincide with the economic fallout following the Great Recession.[28] We do know that mental health problems are increasing more generally in this age group, and we do know that young girls are using more lethal methods when they attempt suicide, therefore they are more likely to die.[29] We also know that child and adolescent mental health services are under huge pressures, that there are long waiting lists for treatment and that, in some countries, their funding has been cut year-on-year since the 2008 recession. All of these factors will be in the mix when the explanation for the increase in young female suicide is eventually uncovered. In the meantime, we must be vigilant and focus our efforts on trying to better understand the nature of the associated risk, who may be at particular risk and what we can do to mitigate the risk. We also ignore potential benefits at our peril, as social media isn't going away anytime soon, so we should harness it for the good.

### The evidence linking social media use to suicide or self-harm

In the last decade, a number of systematic reviews have been published that have summarised the latest research about the nature and extent of the relationship between social media use and different indicators of suicide risk including suicidal ideation, self-harm and suicide attempts.[30] Very little research, however, has investigated the direct relationship between social media use and suicide itself. Most of the reviews have extrapolated their conclusions from suicide attempts or self-harm to suicide.

When considering the relationship between social media use and suicide attempts or self-harm, it is important to investigate potential benefits as well as potential harms. One of the reviews published in 2020 was by Candice Biernesser and colleagues from the University of Pittsburgh, which focused on 24 of the highest quality studies that had investigated social media use and suicide risk in young people.[31] Unsurprisingly, those young people who were defined as heavy or problematic users of social media were more likely to report suicidal ideation or behaviour. They also found evidence that cyberbullying and rejection were associated with suicidal thoughts, self-harm and suicide attempts in young people from different countries. This latter finding builds upon a review led by Ann John, from Swansea University, who found that compared to those who had not been victims of cyberbullying, those who had experienced cybervictimisation were more than twice as likely to self-harm or to attempt suicide.[32]

There was also some evidence that seeking out information about suicide or self-harm online was associated with suicide risk. Young people who were suicidal also had stronger social media linkages with others who were similarly suicidal. In many ways these findings are to be expected, and we need to be careful not to draw conclusions about cause and effect as these relationships are only associations. Having said that, in one of the studies, adolescents who had self-harmed did say that seeing other people's images of self-harm influenced their own self-harm. As a result, it is welcome that social media platforms such as Instagram have introduced new safeguarding rules, which include removing potentially triggering content. As always, however, there is a fine line between safeguarding and perceived censorship as some young people feel that the removal of self-harm images serves only to add to the stigma that they feel. But I believe, on balance, as exposure can act as a volitional moderator, we need to curb exposure to such imagery in online spaces.

Biernesser's review also focused on the benefits of social media use for young people. In five of the studies, social media provided social support and a sense of connectedness, which is protective. For example, although some young people reported negative exchanges on social media, many of the exchanges were supportive, offering the young people empathy and helping them to manage their own emotional pain. There were also examples of social support being provided via social media as well as instances of signposting for young people to self-harm or suicide prevention resources. Overall then, it is clear that there are risks associated with social media, especially for those young people who are already vulnerable, but a measured approach to understanding the role of social media in suicide risk is required. Moreover, we've seen that social media has its benefits and can be harnessed to help rather than hinder young people.

## Media representations

In the late nineties, I remember being surprised by the findings of an intriguing study that showed that people's likelihood of self-harm could be influenced by what they had watched on television. In this case, the researchers were interested in the portrayal of an intentional overdose during an episode of the British medical drama *Casualty*.[33] They wanted to see whether there was a rise in cases of overdose across the UK after the episode was broadcast. The findings were pretty clear. There was a 17 per cent increase in self-poisonings to hospitals in the week following the initial broadcast. In addition, when a sub-sample of those who had taken an overdose were interviewed, 20 per cent said that watching the episode had influenced their decision to self-harm.

Now, if we fast forward to 2017, Netflix released the phenomenally successful TV show *13 Reasons Why*.[34] The series revolves around the suicide of Hannah Baker, a teenage girl, and the '13 reasons' why she took her life. Immediately after its initial streaming, I, and countless others involved in suicide prevention, was concerned that it might spark suicidal contagion, especially in young people. The furore led to Netflix adding an additional warning to the show's broadcast. Our concern was that the show breached the international media reporting guidelines around suicide. These guidelines are not trying to censor programme-makers; rather they are trying to promote responsible and ethical reporting of suicide in the media.[35] They provide practical advice such as not to give unnecessary details of suicide method or location of death, to avoid sensational headlines, not to provide simplistic explanations for suicide and to promote messages of recovery.

Specifically, in the final episode, the coverage of Hannah's suicide was graphic and gratuitous, which is contrary to the guidelines not to provide detailed depictions of a method of death. As I wrote in a blog at the time, the portrayal of Hannah's suicide as inevitable and that suicide was the only option was unhelpful.[36] An implicit message was also that help-seeking does not get you anywhere and I felt that the aftermath of the suicide was also glamorised. A study covering the three months after the initial release of *13 Reasons Why* has reinforced our fears.[37] Although the authors of the study urged caution in interpreting their findings, they found a 12 per cent and a 22 per cent increase in 10–19-year-old male and female suicides respectively in the period immediately after streaming began. A subsequent study also reported increases in the overall suicide rates in 10–17-year-olds in the US.[38] However, there has been some debate since about the analyses used in the latter study.[39] But there were also some findings from a survey of adolescents and parents in the US, UK, Brazil, Australia and New Zealand, conducted by Northwestern University and commissioned by Netflix, that focused on some potential benefits.[40] According to this report, the show has prompted discussions between parents and their children about difficult topics such as suicide, mental health and bullying. Irrespective of this debate, thankfully, Netflix has now removed the offending scene depicting Hannah's death. Programme-makers need to be mindful of their responsibilities.

The relationship between media exposure and suicidal behaviour is not limited to television. It extends to news reporting of suicide, especially the coverage of suicide by celebrities.[41] The influence of the media depiction of suicide or self-harm on triggering suicidal behaviour in others is often called the 'Werther effect'.[42] It is so called after the suicide of the protagonist in Goethe's novel *The Sorrows of Young Werther*, who took his life after being rejected by the woman he loved. When this novel was published in 1774, there were reports from across Europe of young men killing themselves using the same method, as if being influenced by reading the book and identifying with Young Werther. Such suicides are sometimes called copycat or imitative suicides or described as cases of suicidal contagion.

Since the term the Werther effect was first coined in the seventies, numerous studies and reviews have concluded that there is clear evidence that media depictions of suicide are associated with increases in fatal and non-fatal suicidal behaviour. The effects are not as strong as many other risk factors and tend to be short-lived. To get an idea of the scale of the impact of media reporting of suicide, Thomas Niederkrotenthaler from the Medical University of Vienna, Austria, together with Matt Spittal from Melbourne University and others, examined all relevant studies since the Second World War.[43] This is the most comprehensive review conducted to date, and it focused on celebrity suicides. They found that the risk of suicide increased by 13 per cent in the immediate time period, usually a month after the media reporting. These findings are disturbing and they illustrate starkly why the media reporting guidelines around suicide need to be adhered to in full.

More recently, attention has shifted to harnessing media reporting for the good. Niederkrotenthaler has also led the way in this regard, exploring how the media can play a positive role in preventing suicide. To this end, he has coined the term the 'Papageno effect', based on Papageno, a character in Mozart's opera *The Magic Flute* who overcame a suicidal crisis after others showed him different ways of coping.[44] Accordingly, the Papageno effect is defined as the impact of any media reporting that is suicide-protective. For example, it may be beneficial for journalists to report positive outcomes of people who have overcome a suicidal crisis. Such reporting sends out a hopeful message to someone who is in a suicidal crisis that things can get better and that they should hold on. In terms of the IMV model, such messages reduce the deleterious effects of exposure to suicide and may help an individual to feel less trapped and they can disrupt the pathway from suicidal thoughts to suicidal acts. They offer a model that recovery is possible. One of the challenges as we move forward, though, is how we best translate our knowledge of media influences to make the Internet and social media safer places. We need less Werther and more Papageno!

## Suicide clusters

A final concern linked to exposure is what is known as a suicide cluster. This is a group of suicides that occur relatively close together in time or space. There is no agreement, however, about how many suicides comprise a cluster, but it is often interpreted as being more than what would be expected statistically or in a community. Clusters tend to be described as being either 'point' clusters or 'mass' clusters. Point clusters are a group of deaths that occur close together in both time and space, usually within a community or institution over a short period of time, whereas mass clusters are a group of suicides where the deaths happen across the whole population within a relatively brief period of time. The increases in deaths following a celebrity suicide would be a case of a mass cluster. A group of suicides in a school in the same term might be a point cluster. Arguably, things are even more difficult to define in the age of the Internet and social media.

Jo Robinson, Jane Pirkis and I wrote a chapter on suicide clusters for *The International Handbook of Suicide Prevention* that reviews the key issues related to clusters.[45] For example, suicide clusters are much rarer than people think, with estimates ranging from 1 to 10 per cent of all suicides, depending on the population or setting. They are more common among young people and in schools or psychiatric units. In terms of why clusters occur, there are at least two explanations. The first is suicidal contagion and imitation, whereby individuals who are exposed to the suicide of someone else model that behaviour. This is more likely to happen if they identify with the person who has died in some way. The second is called assortative relating or susceptibility and it describes when a group of suicides occur because high-risk individuals associate with each other in a specific setting such as a hospital. Thomas Joiner from Florida State University found that this assortative effect extended to college students, with those students who chose to room together (roommates) being more similar on a suicide index than those who were assigned a room together.[46] Although relatively rare, more needs to be done to ensure individuals, communities and institutions are vigilant and act proactively to minimise the risk of clusters occurring.

## Impulsivity

Impulsivity is the fourth volitional factor associated with the transition from suicidal thoughts to suicidal acts. Despite it being part of our everyday discourse, there are many different definitions of impulsivity and different modes of assessment that complicate our understanding of the impulsivity–suicide risk relationship. For the present purposes, I'm using the term 'impulsivity' to describe a personality trait that is characterised by the tendency to act rashly, without thinking through the consequences of one's actions. The associated logic pertaining to why it is a volitional moderator is relatively straightforward. If someone is thinking about ending their life and they tend to act impulsively, then it stands to reason that they are more likely to act on their thoughts than someone who isn't impulsive. Like many risk factors for suicide, however, the strength and nature of the relationship is up for debate and, in some cases, impulsivity is not implicated in suicidal behaviour at all, with the suicide being very carefully planned.[47]

To untangle the impulsivity–suicide risk relationship, it is also useful to distinguish between the impulsivity of an individual and the impulsivity of the suicidal act. Suicidal behaviour can result if someone acts impulsively, although it can also happen if someone is very deliberate by nature but the act itself is impulsive. The strength of the relationship between impulsivity and suicide risk is also likely to vary across the lifespan. Specifically, as levels of impulsivity are thought to peak in our mid-twenties, the relative influence of impulsivity on suicide risk is likely to diminish as we get older. When considering impulsivity, we also need to factor in the effect of other disinhibiting factors such as alcohol, drugs and lack of sleep. Each of these factors may contribute to an impulsive suicidal act irrespective of your trait impulsivity.

Across a number of research studies we have compared impulsivity in people who have thought about suicide but who have never attempted suicide and in those who have attempted suicide.[48] Time and again, consistent with the IMV model, we have found the same thing: people who have attempted suicide report higher levels of impulsivity than those who have only thought about it. However, the strength of the association between impulsivity and suicidal behaviour varies across studies, with some studies finding a small association. To complicate matters further, more recent research, including some of our own, has found that a particular aspect of impulsivity – negative urgency – is more centrally involved in the transition from suicidal thoughts to suicide attempts.[49] Negative urgency is an emotion-based type of impulsivity that comprises acting rashly when in a negative or distressed state. In the context of suicide risk this makes sense, because negative urgency is also associated with impairments in self-regulation, specifically in our capacity to inhibit our impulses. If you rate highly on negative urgency and you also feel trapped, it may be more difficult to inhibit the urge to act on your suicidal thoughts and therefore suicidal behaviour becomes more likely. We have also found that alcohol-related negative urgency is perhaps unsurprisingly associated with the transition from thoughts to suicidal acts.[50]

## Physical Pain Sensitivity

Physical pain sensitivity and fearlessness about death are often grouped together into one subheading because, as I noted in the previous chapter, they comprise Thomas Joiner's concept of capability for suicide.[51] Indeed, there is little disagreement that capability is important in the transition from thoughts to acts of suicide. However, in terms of the IMV model, I believe that capability is only one of a number of volitional factors that governs behavioural enaction, whereas within Joiner's interpersonal theory, capability is seen as the key factor to determine whether someone acts on their suicidal thoughts or not. David Klonsky, a psychologist from the University of British Columbia, also takes a wider perspective on capability. In his three-step theory of suicide, he argues that there are three categories of variables that contribute to the capability of suicide:[52]

1. dispositional (e.g., genetic factors such as pain sensitivity)
2. acquired (e.g., habituation to pain)
3. practical (e.g., having access to the means of suicide)

The three-step theory alongside the IMV model and Joiner's interpersonal theory are often referred to as ideation-to-action models as they focus on the transition from suicidal thoughts to suicidal acts.[53] Irrespective of theoretical perspective, however, a wide range of studies has shown that physical pain sensitivity and fearlessness about death are associated with suicidal behaviour and differentiate between suicidal thoughts and suicide attempts, with people who attempt suicide being able to tolerate higher levels of physical pain and being less fearful of dying than those who have only thought about suicide.[54]

I know I've mentioned physical pain sensitivity several times, but I haven't described how it is measured. You may not be surprised to learn that it is tricky to assess the extent to which we are sensitive to physical pain or how much pain we can tolerate. Some researchers (including me) use self-report questionnaires that ask respondents to rate how painful they find things, but personally I find such questions very difficult to answer.[55] And that is despite having my own unplanned-for encounter with physical pain: In my first year at university I smashed my knee-cap on an evening out but luckily I managed to make my way to the local emergency department without fainting and with a little help from my friends (don't ask, but it involved misplaced hubris in a concrete bollard jumping competition, an extended stay in hospital in the lead-up to Christmas in 1991 and having to learn to walk again!). Therefore, I think I have pretty good pain tolerance. Nonetheless, I still find it difficult to rate my own sensitivity or tolerance to physical pain on a self-report measure. As a result, I am not particularly confident in the accuracy of asking people how sensitive they are to pain as a way of measuring their physical pain tolerance.

More recently, therefore, we have moved away from asking people about their physical pain sensitivity to using more experimental methods to assess physical pain threshold and tolerance. We tend to use an algometer, a pressure gauge rigged up to a computer, that allows us to record the pressure or force that is exerted, usually to the palm of the hand, under different experimental conditions.[56] It gives us a more direct measure of pain sensitivity and tolerance. In such studies, we record the pressure that is induced in Pascals, rather than pain per se, but as the experience can be briefly uncomfortable it is thought to be analogous to the experience of pain. The safety and well-being of participants is always our number one priority, so, of course, all participants provide informed consent in advance about the nature of the study and there are no residual effects of the algometer. They are also able to withdraw from a given study at any time without giving a reason.

The general practice across such experimental studies is that we exert pressure (or the participant exerts pressure themselves) to the palm of the participant's hand via the algometer and record when they tell us that the pressure/force starts to feel uncomfortable. This gives us a measure of their pain threshold. Then we exert increasing amounts of pressure and ask participants to tell us when they have had enough and we use this level as an indicator of their pain tolerance. Such studies allow us to investigate whether pain tolerance differs by suicidal history, whether it changes over time and if tolerance is higher in someone who is feeling down, trapped or stressed. The logic surrounding why people who are suicidal can tolerate higher levels of physical pain tolerance is as follows:

- People who are suicidal are so overwhelmed by emotional pain (e.g., when trapped) that their capacity to perceive physical pain is reduced.
- This allows them to tolerate higher levels of physical pain than usual, without experiencing it as so painful to be aversive.
- If they can tolerate higher levels of physical pain, then they may be able to withstand the pain associated with a potentially more painful and potentially more lethal suicidal act.

This type of research is intriguing, but it is still in its infancy. It is important though as it helps us to understand crucial processes that may underpin suicidal acts, and that unlocking these doors will allow us to save lives. Olivia Kirtley, Ronan O'Carroll and I reviewed all of the studies on pain sensitivity and self-harm and, although there is definitely a relationship, there are still so many unanswered questions about the nature of this relationship.[57] For example, is physical pain tolerance the same in people who cut themselves without suicidal intent compared to those who attempt suicide? Or how does physical pain tolerance relate to people who engage in less physically painful suicidal behaviour? Or how does repeated self-harm affect physical pain tolerance? Or do gender differences in pain sensitivity account, in part, for the differences in suicide rates in men and women? Olivia has also extended these questions to understanding suicidal ideation and behaviour in individuals with chronic pain.[58]

Despite the fact that we have so much more to learn, this type of research is a good example of a novel approach to investigating who is more likely to cross the precipice, to attempt suicide when they are experiencing suicidal thoughts. Sadly though, we are nowhere near the point where we can say a specific level of physical pain tolerance is associated with a particular level of suicide risk.

## Fearlessness about Death

It is often said that in order to end one's life we have to overcome the fundamental instinct to live. Beyond biological preparedness, I don't know whether such an instinct exists in a conscious way, but the life instinct ('eros') was one of the basic instincts espoused by Sigmund Freud in his essay *Beyond the Pleasure Principle* published in the 1920s, the other being the death drive ('thanatos').[59] Freud believed that human life is characterised by a struggle between these two forces. According to psychoanalysts, suicide results when the death drive is in the ascendency and the aggression associated with thanatos is directed inward. Indeed, consistent with this approach, Karl Menninger, the American psychiatrist, talked about suicide as being murder in the 180th degree.[60] Irrespective of the psychodynamic underpinnings, however, to kill oneself is ostensibly an aggressive act, directed at the self, and by definition it requires one to overcome an innate fear of dying to some degree, at least.

As noted above, fearlessness about death – the sixth volitional factor – is the second component of the capability for suicide. There is clear evidence from studies conducted over many years that people who have attempted suicide report less fear about suicide and dying itself more generally than those who haven't attempted suicide.[61] Fearlessness about death is a cognitive factor that is more amenable to assessment by self-report than physical pain sensitivity. Indeed, a few years ago, Jessica Ribeiro and colleagues developed the ACSS-Fearlessness about Death scale (ACSS-FAD).[62] This seven-item scale asks respondents to endorse the extent to which items such as 'The fact that I am going to die does not affect me' and 'I am not at all afraid to die' are like or not like them on a five-point rating scale. Those who score more highly on these items, and who are also suicidal, are more likely to act on their thoughts of suicide than those who score lower on this scale, and are therefore at greater risk of suicide as a consequence. If a loved one is talking about being trapped and how they are not frightened of dying, respond quickly to check that they feel safe and that they are not going to act on any thoughts of suicide.

In our research, we have also shown that people who have attempted suicide are less fearful of dying than those who have only thought about suicide. For example, in the Scottish Well-being Study, led by my colleagues Karen Wetherall and Seonaid Cleare, we surveyed 3,500 young adults living in Scotland, and we asked them to answer a range of questions about their mental health. In one of the first academic papers that we published from this study, we compared respondents with different suicidal histories on a whole range of psychological factors including fearlessness about death.[63] When we did the analyses, consistent with the IMV model and Thomas Joiner's interpersonal theory, those who had attempted suicide were markedly less fearful of dying than those who had only thought about suicide. Even more striking though, this difference in fearlessness about dying didn't seem to be explained by different levels of depression or entrapment. This is important to note because it suggests that it isn't simply that those who have attempted suicide are more depressed than those who have only thought about it. It also serves as a reminder that the transition from suicidal thoughts to suicidal acts is largely governed by volitional factors.

Here's Stan, whom I met in one of my clinical studies, who had attempted suicide after an 'awful' time in his life when his world 'fell apart' in his mid-thirties. He talked about how his fear of dying (fearlessness about death) had changed over time:

It was just one thing after another. It seemed to be never-ending. First, I lost my job in the shipyard, then my wee brother died. Both happened last February. I still cannot believe he's gone. We were best mates. I was really angry, just angry with everyone and anyone. I was picking fights with any Tom, Dick or Harry; drinking, sleeping, and fighting. Then one night, I was off my face, I'd had enough and I just hated myself. I just wanted to end it all, but I just couldn't do it. I was shit-scared. I'd thought of doing myself in a while back as well, when my wife left me, but then it passed; I didn't really think that much about it then or what I'd do. But since Mikey's gone, I couldn't give a shit any more. So, I'd wake up in the morning, and it's like all I'd think about. And the more I thought about it, the more I thought 'what is there to be frightened about?', 'sure I'll be dead', 'what's the problem, as long as I do it right?'. And I promised myself that the next time the shit hits the fan, that's it. And I kept my promise, but I cannot believe I am still here.

Stan was so angry, but my memory of meeting him is that, despite his anger, he wasn't being aggressive. He was just being very matter-of-fact. I wish I had asked him directly why or how his fear of dying had changed, because it clearly had. Halfway through he talks about being 'shit-scared', which I took to mean scared of dying. Then, later on, after being preoccupied with suicide for a while, he seems to have had some sort of 'breakthrough', as if something changed or shifted such that he was no longer frightened to die. This could have been exhaustion or a consequence of his anger. It's as if he had worked out in his head what he would do (in terms of method) and what the outcome would be (death). It is also not clear what the timeline for the shift was; did he overcome his fearfulness quickly or did it take time, and what triggered the shift in thinking? I'll never know. I sometimes wonder whether he is still alive or not.

Stan's story illustrates another challenge in suicide prevention. We need to better understand what makes someone less fearful about dying. Is it that the more exposure we have to dying and death the more we become fearless? Is fearlessness related to risk-taking or is it a by-product of rock-bottom self-esteem or mental exhaustion? Could it be that the fear of living is more painful than the fear of dying? There are so many unanswered questions. We also need to disentangle the extent to which other volitional factors interact to affect fearlessness about death. Once again, as we make advances in our understanding of suicide risk, they uncover more and more new questions.

## Mental Imagery

I'd spend days thinking about being dead. But it was more than that – I could picture myself being dead. I was back at my mum and dad's and it was really vivid, like in technicolour, like I was actually there . . .

These words from Mo, who attempted suicide in his mid-fifties, eloquently illustrate one aspect of mental imagery: visualising oneself after death. This type of mental imagery is an example of visual imagery, although mental imagery can involve any of our five senses. Mental imagery about dying or death is the penultimate volitional factor. Some people who attempt suicide or who have subsequently died by suicide also report experiencing images of actually dying by their own hand, while carrying out the suicidal act, as if they're in the heat of the moment. In terms of suicide risk, the concern is that mental imagery, a cognitive volitional factor, forms part of the rehearsal process that precedes a suicidal act. Like any other type of rehearsal, the replaying in our mind's eye, of any behaviour, increases the likelihood that we'll enact that behaviour.

Take the use of mental imagery by athletes as an illustration. There is a large body of research evidence showing that mental imagery improves their performance.[64] I am most definitely not an athlete, but I play a lot of tennis and I am always thinking of new ways to improve my game. So I often turn to self-help books and, without exception, they all focus on mental imagery as a key technique to optimise your game. They'll instruct you to picture the ball going over the net or your execution of the perfect backhand, landing the ball deep in your opponent's side of the court. Although I am not sure how useful these techniques are for me, they have been shown to be effective and the same principles hold for other behaviours, including for suicidal behaviour. These mental images, similar to those of Mo's, may also increase suicide risk by making us less fearful about dying. If you consider the first time someone thinks about or pictures themselves dying, it may elicit a physiological response; a bit like a fight or flight response – their heart rate may increase or they may sweat. This response may also include feeling anxious or frightened and as a result they may be put off carrying out the act. However, the next time such an image comes to mind, perhaps they become less frightened and, over time, they may habituate to being exposed to such images and as a result they become less fearful about dying. And if they're less fearful their suicide risk increases. Indeed, in the Scottish Wellbeing Study we found that people who had attempted suicide reported higher levels of mental imagery about their death than those who had only thought about suicide.[65] We assess mental imagery using a measure developed by Emily Holmes, a clinical psychologist working in

Sweden.[66] This measure asks people to imagine death-related imagery when they feel down or distressed, including engaging in self-harm or suicide. For example, one of the questions asks people how often they picture images of themselves planning/preparing to self-harm or make a suicide attempt.

Emily also talks about particular types of suicide-related imagery as 'flash-forwards'. These flash-forwards are so-called because they are images that relate to potentially future suicidal thoughts or acts. They are thought to be akin to flashbacks often reported in individuals with post-traumatic stress disorder, who experience intrusive and vivid images about a past traumatic event. Flash-forwards also tend to be imbued with a sense of reality, being rich in detail. Those experiencing them also report being more preoccupied with these images than with verbal thoughts about suicide. These characteristics fit with Mo's description of his suicidal images as being 'in technicolour, like I was actually there'. These images are also often rated as being both distressing and comforting. This is not that surprising, as we know that ambivalence often characterises thoughts of suicide.[67] But the feelings of comfort may be rewarding for the individual, and this reinforcement may make it more likely that these images 'pop' back into our mind again and again. There is also one study from Hong Kong that has shown that entrapment when experienced alongside suicidal flash-forwards predicts worse suicidal thoughts.[68]

The take-home message, therefore, is that mental imagery about suicide may increase the likelihood of someone acting on their thoughts of suicide, so targeting these flash-forwards in treatment may be a fruitful aim to prevent suicide. In other words, if someone is picturing themselves dying or dead, they could benefit from some help to address the content of these images to make it less likely that they'll act on them. Indeed, led by Martina Di Simplicio, Emily and colleagues have recently tested a novel brief imagery-based psychological intervention called Imaginator in young people who self-harm.[69] Their initial feasibility study is promising, suggesting that it may help young people reduce self-harm, but a full RCT is required to determine whether it works. Finally, similar to the unanswered questions around the capability of suicide, we don't know yet how the mental imagery about dying and death develops.

## Past Suicidal Behaviour

The eighth and final volitional factor is arguably the most important because we know that if someone crosses the precipice from thoughts to acts of suicide once, they are more likely to do so again. Put simply and as I've said elsewhere, past suicidal behaviour is one of the best predictors of future suicidal behaviour.[70] Despite the latter statement being scientifically accurate, however, I need to add two caveats:

1. You may remember that, earlier in this book, I said that our ability to predict suicide is no better than chance, no more accurate than the toss of a coin.[71] This is true. Nonetheless, it still doesn't prevent a past history of suicide attempts or self-harm being one of the single best predictors of suicide. Statistically speaking, if you engage in suicidal behaviour once, then you are more likely to do so again. And it doesn't seem to make a difference whether the past self-injurious behaviour was suicidal in intent (suicide attempt) or not (non-suicidal self-harm).[72] Take all acts of self-injurious behaviour seriously.

2. Statistical risk isn't the same as clinical risk. Do you remember the section on the difference between absolute versus relative risk from earlier (page 154)? Relative risk can sound really scary even when the absolute risk is relatively low. It is important to hold on to the fact that the vast majority of people who engage in suicidal behaviour will never attempt suicide or self-harm again, nor will they end their life by suicide. So, the absolute risk of suicide is low. In our clinical studies, between 20 and 30 per cent of people who are admitted to hospital following a suicide attempt are treated again for another suicide attempt within 12 months and very much fewer than 1 per cent will die by suicide.[73]

Recently, epidemiologists from David Gunnell's suicide and self-harm research group at the University of Bristol reviewed all of the research evidence related to repeated self-harm and subsequent suicide among patients who had previously presented to hospital with self-harm.[74] This allowed them to quantify the risk of suicide and they found that 1 in 25 patients who presented to hospital following self-harm died by suicide within 5 years. In addition, 16 per cent of these patients engaged in another episode of self-harm within 12 months. This repeat self-harm figure is lower than in some of our studies because our studies tend to include more medically serious suicide attempts. The key message, therefore, is that the vast majority of people who have a history of suicidal behaviour will never attempt suicide again or die by suicide. But it is important for us not to be complacent – even though we cannot predict suicide particularly well, we should always be thinking about what we can do to keep everyone who has a suicidal history safe.

## Using the IMV Model to Understand Suicide Risk

When Olivia Kirtley and I updated the IMV model in 2018, in addition to better defining the volitional phase of the model, we also added dotted lines to each of the figures (Figures 1 and 2) to recognise the dynamic and cyclical relationship between suicidal ideation and suicidal behaviour.[75]

For some people, they can become caught in a temporal cycle of thinking about suicide, acting on their thoughts, back to feeling trapped and then once again experiencing suicidal thoughts and perhaps engaging in another suicide attempt. For others, sadly, they die by suicide on their first attempt. Although it is difficult to accurately quantify how many people kill themselves on their first attempt, the best evidence suggests that more than half will do so.[76] This is a heartbreaking statistic that highlights the importance of early intervention and the need to intervene before someone gets to the stage of attempting suicide, because, for the majority, it will end in death. As a consequence, we need to focus our suicide prevention efforts on those individual, social and cultural factors that lead to defeat, humiliation, loss, shame, rejection and entrapment. We also need to recognise the dynamic interplay of different risk factors to maximise our suicide prevention efforts. Indeed, my friend and colleague Ellen Townsend, a psychologist from the University of Nottingham, has developed a card sort task – the Card Sort Task for Self-harm (CaTS) – that helps to map out the patterns of thoughts, feelings, behaviours and events that lead to self-harm.[77] With such an approach, it is possible to depict the relative influence of risk factors for different self-harm episodes and tailor interventions to different people. Not only does the CaTS allow us to explore directly which specific factors are related to someone's self-harm or suicide attempt, it helps us to identify chains of sequences of factors. For example, it could be that self-hatred led to feelings of anger, that led to worthlessness, which in turn led to feelings of entrapment – and then entrapment led to the suicidal behaviour. With such detailed information, it may be possible to pre-empt a subsequent crisis escalating or it could point to factors that could be targeted with clinical interventions. If you notice these patterns of thoughts, emotions and behaviours developing, you may want to check in with a loved one to see if they need help or support. It may also be possible to use this information as an early warning system highlighting that someone could benefit from professional support.

While recognising that the circumstances surrounding every death by suicide are unique, as described above, the IMV model endeavours to illuminate the common factors and pathways that can lead to suicide. If we consider the volitional phase, I don't expect all eight volitional factors to be involved in all suicide attempts or every death by suicide. However, I would use the details outlined in Figure 2 to systematically explore the likelihood that someone will act on their thoughts of suicide. It may be that they have a plan in place for a particular method of death; and if this is the case I'd focus efforts on ensuring the environment is safe. Indeed, this is the focus of the next part.

Before closing this chapter, I'd like to use a more detailed vignette of someone who died by suicide, to further illustrate some of the pathways to suicide. As I've done elsewhere in the book, this example is based on someone, Paul, who took his own life, but some of the details have been changed to maintain confidentiality. By working through Paul's vignette, hopefully it will become clearer how the IMV model can be useful in understanding suicide risk and thinking through how it may apply to someone you may be concerned about. In addition, if you are a mental health professional it will illustrate how the IMV model can serve as a framework to formulate a treatment plan around someone who is vulnerable.

Paul was 54 when he died. His mother had a history of alcoholism and, although he described himself as an everyday drinker, he rarely got excessively drunk. He worked in IT. His first marriage ended four years prior to his death. He had two children and had embarked on a new relationship with someone he had known since his childhood days. Following the breakdown of his marriage, he had moved jobs to another part of the country. He moved back to where he had grown up, but he hadn't lived there since his student days. The new relationship didn't last long, ending 18 months after it began. He had become pretty isolated. Despite having a good relationship with his children, they were both at university in other parts of the country and they were busy leading their own lives.

As a teenager, Paul had suffered from low mood and had been hospitalised for self-harm, but he had never been formally diagnosed with depression and had never been prescribed medication for mental health problems. His uncle, whom he had been close to as a child, had taken his own life a couple of years previously and Paul had taken the death very badly. According to his eldest son, he felt alone and was always his own harshest critic, and not long before his death he had become quite emotionally flat, saying that he wasn't surprised that he was on his own as he was 'no longer of any use to anyone' and his life had amounted to nothing. He also regretted that he had not stayed in touch with his university friends.

Sadly, Paul's story is not that unusual: a middle-aged divorced man, living alone, takes his own life. In most countries of the world, the majority of people who die by suicide were 'never married', were 'previously married' or were 'single' at the time of death. Middle-aged men in the UK are most at risk of dying by their own hand compared to other age groups.[78] On the face of it, Paul's life story could be that of millions of people, especially if we bear in mind that almost half of all first marriages in the UK end in divorce. That's a lot of people potentially at risk of suicide. So, what was different in Paul's case? Although we can never know for certain why Paul took his own life, we can try to piece together some of the potential contributory factors. In the table below, I have tried to do this very simply in terms of the three parts of the IMV model:

| Pre-motivational phase | Motivational phase | Volitional phase |
| --- | --- | --- |
| • Self-critical<br>• Mother's history of alcoholism<br>• Marriage breakdown and end of new relationship | • Lack of social support<br>• Thwarted belonging<br>• No longer any use to anyone<br>• Lack of any future thoughts<br>• Feelings of defeat and entrapment | • Past history of self-harm<br>• Exposure to suicide of uncle |

When using the IMV model as a framework to try to make sense of a suicide, I consider the extent to which an individual may have felt defeated or humiliated, and whether they were in a situation from which they perceived there to be no escape. As I have said repeatedly, entrapment, the *perception* of being trapped, is so pernicious because it is this perception that drives so much suicidal distress. Obviously, I'd also try to piece together any relevant life history. What (if any) vulnerability did an individual carry with them, and was this exacerbated by negative life events in the days, weeks or months before they died? In Paul's case, there seem to have been several red flags from his distant and more recent past that are likely to have contributed to his suicide risk.

Let's start with the pre-motivational phase of the IMV model. You will remember that this phase attempts to determine the background context and negative life events that may have contributed to or triggered the suicide or suicide attempt, or were the straws that broke the camel's back. Paul's son talks about him being his 'own harshest critic', which may point to high levels of self-criticism. Self-criticism is a personality trait and vulnerability factor that is associated with poor mental health and suicidal ideation.[79] Crucially, though, its negative effect is most marked under periods of stress. In and of itself, self-criticism does not lead to suicide, but it can increase the likelihood that someone feels defeated. It can also drive the ruminative thoughts associated with depression, hopelessness and entrapment.[80] It acts a bit like socially prescribed perfectionism that I discussed earlier (page 114).

As we've seen, understanding one's environment and the experience of negative life events, including early life trauma, are important. We don't know much about Paul's environment beyond the note that his mother had a history of alcoholism. This may have had an adverse impact on Paul's well-being during his childhood and affected the development of attachment relationships. Sadly, the greater the exposure to such ACEs, the more the increase in the likelihood of poor mental and physical health outcomes in adulthood, including of suicide attempts and suicide.[81]

The comment about being 'no longer of any use to anyone' is also potentially linked to Paul feeling that he was a burden on others (his children) and this, together with him thinking that his life had not amounted to anything, will have contributed to his feelings of defeat. In his depressed state he may have been unable to see any hope and, despite having children, he still felt alone and was lacking in social support. Again, Paul's circumstances are lived out, up and down the country, each and every day. Middle-aged men who have invested the bulk of their emotional support eggs in the single basket of their life partner are at increased risk of being socially isolated if this relationship breaks down.[82]

In terms of the volitional phase, Paul had history. He had at least two specific markers that may have contributed to his transition from suicidal thoughts to the fatal suicidal act. Although it was many years ago, he had self-harmed in the past, and at least one of the episodes was of sufficient medical severity to have resulted in hospitalisation. So he would have known that he had the capability to self-harm again. Perhaps his previous thoughts of self-injury were reignited when his uncle took his life, which he had taken badly, and then, when this is added to his sense of social isolation, hopelessness and entrapment, he had just had enough. Being mentally exhausted, he took things into his own hands and ended the pain by taking his own life.

Paul's death illustrates a key premise of the IMV model. It highlights that for suicide to occur it requires both the motivation (thoughts of suicide) and the volition (factors that make someone act on their thoughts of suicide). It also helps us to think about where we might intervene to prevent a future Paul dying by suicide. The model highlights that we can intervene both at the motivational phase and the volitional phase, as intervention at both levels can reduce the likelihood that someone attempts or dies by suicide. As I said earlier, although it is difficult to predict each individual suicide, the IMV model should help any one of us to think about risk and potential protective factors in those around us. So, when we are thinking about helping someone, we can consider intervening at the motivational phase to stop the emergence of thoughts of suicide as well as interventions aimed at the volitional phase, that are focused on stopping someone acting on their thoughts of suicide. I return to the topic of helping someone who is vulnerable in the remaining chapters of this book. I will provide practical advice about the potentially daunting task of asking someone about suicide, as well as describing ways of keeping people who are vulnerable safe. I will also take you through how best to help individuals who are supporting people who are suicidal as well as those trying to survive the aftermath of suicide.

# Part 3

# What Works to Keep People Who Are Suicidal Safe

I will never forget being told that my close friend Clare had died. That telephone call. It is a moment frozen in time, a flashbulb memory, vivid and painful. I remember the tears, the shock; it was impossible to fathom. When I close my eyes and think about Clare, I am transported right back to that awful moment of discovery, and to the guilt and the questions about what else I could have done. She had seemed fine, she was in a good place when I had last spoken to her, and her final email, a few days beforehand, hadn't rung any alarm bells for me. The previous few months had been tough for her, but I thought Clare was much happier and that she could see the light at the end of the tunnel. My experience is not uncommon, and many friends, partners, parents and children will have gone through the very same, asking themselves why they were not able to keep those close to them safe. What else could or should they have done? Of course, we cannot bring back our loved ones, but we may be able to help others in the future, whether we are clinicians, researchers, family members, friends or colleagues.

In this part, I will take you through some of the interventions that have been shown to be effective in terms of trying to support people at risk of suicide. Intervention is a term to describe a strategy, a technique, a tool or some other component or components that is designed to bring about a change in behaviour or health status. For the present purposes, the interventions that I discuss here are targeting the reduction or elimination of suicidal thoughts and behaviour. Some of the interventions are longer-term clinical interventions, such as CBT, delivered by trained mental health professionals. Others are briefer and, like safety planning, can be used to help people prepare for and keep themselves safe during difficult times ahead. In Part 4, I will provide further practical information about supporting people who are vulnerable to suicide. Although suicide prevention on an individual level is difficult, if we tackle it head-on, there are things that we can do to reduce the risk. Sadly though, it isn't possible to prevent all suicides, but as a society there is so much more that we can do to prevent these personal tragedies. Suicide prevention must remain a public health imperative.

I begin with an overview of brief interventions before taking you through safety planning, step by step. This part ends with a description of the longer-term interventions that have been shown to work and which offer most promise in terms of alleviating suicidal distress.

# 9

# Brief Contact Interventions

IN CHAPTER 8, I described the Volitional Help Sheet (VHS), one tool that may be helpful to support those who are vulnerable and suicidal, by nudging them away from engaging in a suicidal act (see page 148). But there are a number of other tools like the VHS that have attracted considerable research and clinical attention in recent years that also offer potential avenues of support for people at risk of suicide. These tools are often grouped together as 'brief contact interventions' because, as their name suggests, they are brief in terms of the duration of their delivery and they involve some form of contact with someone who is or has been suicidal. They also do not necessarily need to be delivered by a mental health professional. These types of interventions are different from more longer-term psychological treatments or psychosocial interventions, which I'll discuss in Chapter 11. In these brief interventions the contact can be minimal. For example, it may take the form of receiving a follow-up letter from a clinician or checking in with the person after they have been discharged from hospital. Such approaches have grown in interest in part because too many patients who self-harm or attempt suicide are discharged from hospital with no follow-up care beyond a letter to their GP. They are also helpful for people who do not want to receive ongoing formal outpatient care or who do not seek help in the first place.

Given that such interventions are low in intensity, how might they work? There are a number of different possible explanations for why such brief interventions may be protective. Earlier, I mentioned that receiving a VHS may reduce suicide risk because it activates if-then plans, acting to interrupt the transition from suicidal thoughts to suicidal acts.[1] But that is only one potential mechanism. Low-intensity interventions that focus on maintaining contact with an individual, for example by letter, may also be protective because the simple act of maintaining contact may foster a sense of connectedness, which can be suicide-protective. These letters can also serve as cues for help-seeking, especially if they open the door for someone by simply reminding them that they matter, that they are not a burden and if they are in distress that there is help available. Targeting connectedness and reminding people that they matter make sense as we know from an abundance of research that social disconnection, isolation, thwarted belongingness, shame and feelings of worthlessness all contribute to suicide risk.[2] So, if we can promote connectedness and self-worth, according to the IMV model and the interpersonal theory, that should reduce the likelihood that suicidal thoughts emerge or escalate. Also, we need to consider that some people who present to emergency services following a suicide attempt report negative experiences and leave the emergency department feeling worse than when they arrived.[3] They can feel even more disconnected and dehumanised because they are too often made to feel that they are wasting clinical time and taking up scarce hospital beds. They feel that there are more deserving patients. Although a brief follow-up contact after discharge is no substitute for compassion, dignity and respect when in hospital, it may be one way for someone to feel valued and reminded that their life is worth living and that there is help available. It is important to emphasise that most of the people I have met who deliver frontline clinical services are compassionate and care deeply about the people they treat.

Arguably, the landmark study that kick-started much of the interest in brief contact interventions was published more than 20 years ago by Jerome Motto and Alan Bostrom, both from the University of California, San Francisco.[4] The design of their study was straightforward. Thirty days after discharge from hospital, patients who had been depressed or suicidal but who had not accepted ongoing post-hospital therapy were randomised to receive a brief intervention or not; half of these patients received 'caring letters' and the other half received no further contact. In the caring letters clinicians simply expressed concern for their well-being and invited the recipient to get in touch if they wanted. Here's an example of one of the letters:[5]

Dear John,
It has been some time since you were here at the hospital, and we hope things are going well for you. If you wish to drop us a note we would be glad to hear from you.

These letters were sent monthly for the first four months, then bi-monthly for eight months and then every three months for another four years. In total, therefore, people were sent twenty-four letters over five years. The findings were impressive; over the five years of the study, those who received the letters were less likely to die by suicide compared to those who hadn't received the letters. However, more detailed analyses showed that, although there was benefit across the five years, most of the reduction in suicides was in the first two years of the study. It is worth pausing again to consider the findings. The mere act of maintaining contact with someone who is in distress can have such a powerful suicide-protective effect.

If we translate these findings into our everyday lives, if you think someone is struggling, reach out, drop them a message, check in with them. Sometimes, this may be enough to help them to acknowledge that it is okay not to be okay and to reach out for help. Zahra, who got in touch with me as she was keen to take part in one of our research studies, told me that she thinks she would be dead now if it wasn't for a neighbour checking in on her. She is in her early seventies and lives alone, in a flat, and keeps herself to herself, and would simply exchange pleasantries with her neighbours. However, the previous year had been very difficult for her, as she had lost her only sister and she had endured a period of illness. In her own words, the last year had 'sucked the life out of me'; she had become depressed and had also become quite apprehensive about leaving her flat. She didn't understand why she was worried about going out, but as a result she felt really alone. That winter after her sister had died was marked by so many dark days. She was feeling really low and didn't know whether she could keep going, she was 'quite suicidal'. But then one evening, out of the blue, a neighbour slid a note under her flat door and it simply read, 'How are you doing? I haven't seen you around recently. Hope you're okay. Let me know whether you'd like to meet for a coffee.' That was it. Nothing more, and from someone whom she barely knew – she only knew her to say hello to. She described this simple gesture as 'genuinely life-saving', as it distracted her from her despair briefly. It made her feel valued, and it felt so significant to Zahra because someone had actually taken the time to notice her.

The power of communication is also reflected in the caring letters study. Some of the respondents wrote to the researchers saying that receiving the letters had made them feel valued and connected, similar to Zahra. One of them remarked: 'You will never know what your little notes mean to me. I always think someone cares about what happens to me, even if my family did kick me out. I am really grateful', and another added: 'Your note gave me a warm, pleasant feeling. Just knowing someone cares means a lot.'[6]

Despite these encouraging findings, disappointingly no other caring letters study has demonstrated such an effect on subsequent suicide rates. This is likely, though, to be because most brief intervention studies are not designed to detect changes in suicide rates. Rather, they tend to focus on reducing self-harm or non-fatal suicidal behaviour. Indeed, over the last five to ten years a number of systematic reviews of psychosocial interventions, including brief contact interventions, have been published.[7] Despite applying different criteria, they all point to some benefit of psychosocial interventions. Helpfully, one of these reviews, led by the epidemiologist Allison Milner (who died in a tragic accident in 2019, aged 36), focused specifically on the efficacy of brief contact interventions.[8] It included an evaluation of telephone contacts following presentation to an emergency department or to any healthcare setting, as well as emergency crisis cards and postcard or letter interventions. Crisis cards are sometimes used as part of usual care and are given to patients on discharge and offer crisis admission on-demand or provide some other form of emergency support. The postcard interventions are very similar to the caring letters.

In Milner and colleagues' review, when the findings from the different studies were combined, receiving the brief interventions did not reduce the total number of people who self-harmed or attempted suicide but they did reduce the number of *times* people self-harmed or attempted suicide. You may remember that this was similar to what we found in our VHS study in Scotland.[9] So it may not be possible to stop an individual from engaging in suicidal behaviour entirely, but these brief interventions may help to reduce the frequency of self-harm. If we combine the review findings with our VHS findings, the take-home message is that being supportive is protective. This support can take many different forms including telephone calls, help sheets or letters. Such small acts of support may be especially important when someone does not wish to continue with more formal clinical contact. The more general message for any one of us is that by showing we care we could help to save a life.

# 10

# Safety Planning

MOVING BEYOND BRIEF contact interventions, Stephanie Doupnik and colleagues published another review in 2020.[1] This time they focused on what they described as 'brief acute care suicide prevention interventions', to determine whether they reduced subsequent suicide attempts. Their review included the brief contact interventions discussed in the previous chapter as well as care coordination, safety planning, crisis response planning and other brief therapeutic interventions, such as functional analysis (a way of understanding why a behaviour happens), therapeutic assessment, problem-solving skills and motivational interviewing as well as our VHS. When Doupnik and colleagues synthesised the findings from all studies, they found that these brief acute care suicide prevention interventions were associated with reduced suicide attempts in the weeks and months after discharge from hospital. They also found that those who received these acute interventions were more likely to engage in follow-up mental health care subsequently. Four of the seven studies on suicide attempts had safety planning components, so it is likely that safety planning is driving a significant part of the suicide-protective effect reported. In addition, safety planning has been identified as 'Best Practice' in the joint Suicide Prevention

Resource Centre-American Foundation for Suicide Prevention (SPRC-AFSP) Registry.[2]

Safety planning is a structured intervention co-created usually between a patient and a mental health professional.[3] Its aim is to identify warning signs as well as techniques to help keep someone safe. Put simply, a safety plan is an 'emergency plan' designed to help prevent people from acting on their suicidal feelings. As illustrated in Figure 3 overleaf, a safety plan comprises six steps to be completed by someone, usually after a suicide crisis.[4]

When I first encountered safety planning I must admit to being surprised (in a good way) by its simplicity and its pragmatism. I had heard a lot about safety planning as a technique and I knew that many clinical colleagues were using it in their everyday practice. However, I was also concerned that people were using it in very different ways, with some people giving it to individuals following discharge from hospital and encouraging them to complete it when they got home. This is not best practice as then it isn't possible to talk through their suggestions for each step. Others were working closely and collaboratively with patients, incorporating the safety plan into the patient's ongoing clinical care. This is best practice. I was also conscious, at that stage, that there were no RCTs demonstrating its efficacy in reducing suicidal behaviour. The evidence base has grown since then. Although we are still awaiting the outcomes of a definitive RCT, findings from a wide range of different types of studies confirm that it helps to keep people who are suicidal safe.[6]

Specifically, Barbara Stanley and Gregory Brown, clinical psychologists from the US and the original architects of the safety planning intervention, published a really compelling study in 2018 illustrating the utility of safety planning.[7] In what's called a cohort comparison study, they investigated whether safety

**STEP 1** Warning signs (thoughts, images, mood, situation, behaviour) that a crisis may be developing:

1. ........................................................
2. ........................................................
3. ........................................................

**STEP 2** Internal coping strategies – things I can do to take my mind off my problems without contacting another person (relaxation, physical activity):

1. ........................................................
2. ........................................................
3. ........................................................

**STEP 3** People and social settings that provide distraction:

1. Name: ............ Relationship: ............ Phone: ............
2. Name: ............ Relationship: ............ Phone: ............
3. Place: ........................................................
4. Place: ........................................................

**STEP 4** People who I can ask for help:

1. Name: ............ Relationship: ............ Phone: ............
2. Name: ............ Relationship: ............ Phone: ............
3. Name: ............ Relationship: ............ Phone: ............

**STEP 5** Professionals or agencies I can contact during a crisis:

GP Practice: ............ Phone: ............

GP Name: ........................................................

1. ........................................................
2. ........................................................

**STEP 6** Making the environment safe:

1. ........................................................
2. ........................................................
3. ........................................................

Figure 3. A safety plan[5]

planning together with follow-up telephone contact was associated with reduced suicidal behaviour in patients who had attended veterans' hospital emergency departments in the US. They compared two different sets of hospital sites (the cohort comparison), those in which patients received safety planning and telephone support as well as usual treatment (intervention sites) and those in which patients only received usual treatment (control sites). The findings were extremely positive. There were 45 per cent fewer suicidal behaviours in those sites where patients received the safety planning and telephone support intervention. Compared to the control sites, likelihood of suicidal behaviour over the six months of follow-up was halved in the sites delivering the safety planning plus telephone support. In this study, it was not possible to disentangle the relative influence of the safety plan versus the telephone support. Patients were contacted by telephone at least twice after discharge from hospital and in these calls suicide risk was monitored, patients were given the opportunity to review and revise their safety plan, and barriers to further treatment engagement were explored.

In the UK, we have also conducted a study of safety planning with follow-up telephone support called SAFETEL, to determine whether it is feasible and acceptable to embed the safety planning intervention within the UK NHS.[8] We did so in collaboration with Barbara and Greg, and as part of the study preparation, they trained us in the gold-standard delivery of safety planning. As part of the training, I role-played being a patient who had attempted suicide and Barbara was the mental health professional. This role-play, together with the rest of the training, was incredibly illuminating. It highlighted that safety planning is so much more than the safety planning form. Even though Barbara and I were only role-playing, as we co-created the safety plan, I could sense Barbara's compassion, empathy and warmth. The latter are three cornerstones of safety planning. The safety plan is a tool to help two people to think together about suicidal triggers, to structure ways of mitigating future risk. Its completion is a conversation, a bi-directional dialogue that usually begins with the vulnerable person telling their story of what led them to attempt suicide. In psychology-speak it is vital to be person-centred, to focus on the person in front of you, rather than being protocol-centred and preoccupied with completing the form. It is also important to remember that the person in distress is the expert in their life and in their experiences. I have drawn heavily upon Barbara and Greg's training and the materials that they have developed in this chapter.[9] Their training also highlighted what a safety plan *is* and, perhaps more importantly, what a safety plan *is not*.

A safety plan is designed to act as a short-term intervention to distract an individual from thoughts of suicide until their mood has lifted. Suicidal thoughts wax and wane, they come and go.[10] Therefore the safety plan is integral to keeping someone safe in these moments of acute suicidality, when the thoughts are most prominent. It is difficult to know precisely how long acute suicidal thoughts last for at any one time. They tend to be episodic and of short duration, but for others, they can be more persistent and low-level.[11] For most then, keeping people safe during these short bursts of high-intensity suicidal thoughts is critical to preventing suicidal behaviour. At these moments of potentially imminent risk of suicide, we want to stop the person from crossing from the motivational phase into the volitional phase. My concern is that at such moments the metaphorical door to suicide is open, with the person at risk of walking through it, potentially to their death. This is where the safety plan comes in.

Sticking with the same metaphor, safety planning doesn't close the door per se; rather it distracts the person or it prompts them to contact someone else, or to do something else instead of walking through it. It impedes them from crossing the threshold from suicidal thoughts to a suicidal act and it keeps them safe until the suicidal thoughts subside and the door closes. And when the door reopens, which it will do for many, they are ready. They are prepared to respond once again to keep themselves safe. Put another way, the safety plan enhances an individual's sense of self-control over their suicidal urges and thoughts.

A safety plan is not a tablet set in stone. It is designed to be a dynamic document that may be updated over time. In our SAFETEL study we combined safety planning with follow-up telephone support, similar to what Barbara and Greg had done in the veterans' hospitals. We found that about 20 per cent of people who completed the safety plan in hospital modified their safety plan during the follow-up telephone support.

A safety plan should list internal and social distractions, together with the names and details of people who can be called upon for help in a crisis. Always remember that a safety plan is someone else's plan, it is not your plan. It should be easy to read and written in the person's own words. Doing so should foster a sense of ownership. Crucially, it is a collaboration between two people, usually between a mental health professional and an individual who has been suicidal, and it often fills important gaps in the latter's care or at the end of their care. Barbara and Greg's original impetus behind the development of the safety planning intervention was to keep a person safe in the hiatus between discharge from hospital and follow-up treatment. The collaborative element is fundamental to the effective completion of the safety plan. And the process of collaboration, irrespective of the setting, should convey respect and compassion, which will hopefully help to promote treatment engagement.

The National Collaborating Centre for Mental Health (NCCMH) together with Health Education England (HEE) has developed competency frameworks for self-harm and suicide prevention to enable non-clinicians and clinicians alike to feel confident in delivering a safety plan to anyone who may benefit from it.[12] The frameworks apply to the wider workforce including teachers, youth workers, the police and volunteers, as well as to mental health specialists. They also extend beyond safety planning and highlight the utility of distinguishing between the motivational and volitional phases of suicide risk. I was pleased to be a member of the adult expert reference group who advised on their development as we try to equip the wider community with suicide prevention intervention skills.

Although a risk assessment and a mood check are usually incorporated into the delivery of safety planning, a safety plan is not a long-term tool for mood monitoring or management. It is also not designed for someone at imminent risk of suicide. Remember that if someone is acutely suicidal, standard risk assessment procedures should be followed including contacting emergency services, if necessary. Finally, unless it is adapted and shown to be appropriate, a safety plan should not be used with individuals with cognitive impairment. It is also unclear how feasible standard safety plans are to use with people with different neurodevelopmental profiles, such as autistic people. However, I am involved in a study led by Jacqui Rodgers at Newcastle University in which we are testing the feasibility of an adapted safety plan for autistic individuals.[13] We hope, therefore, that a tailored and effective safety plan will be available for autistic young people soon.

## The Six Steps of Safety Planning

The components that comprise each of the six steps of safety planning are all derived from evidence-based suicide prevention strategies.[14] They include the facilitation of problem-solving and coping skills, the identification and harnessing of social supports, and emergency contacts. They also focus on keeping the environment safe via lethal means restriction, the promotion of service linkage and motivational enhancement to promote community treatment engagement.

Usually a safety plan should be co-developed by a person in distress and a mental health professional. However, if this isn't possible, the following should also help anyone who is supporting someone in crisis to complete a safety plan. In addition to the competency framework mentioned above, 4 Mental Health has also developed really helpful online safety planning resources (see page 279). If you are concerned that someone is at imminent risk of harming themselves, please contact a GP, a mental health professional or the emergency services.

Before completing the safety plan, you should try to obtain an accurate account of the events that transpired before, during and after the most recent suicidal crisis. This description may include the activating or triggering events as well as an individual's reactions to these events. This initial discussion helps to facilitate the identification of warning signs, as well as specific strategies or behaviours that may alleviate the crisis. The safety plan serves as a template to prepare for future risky situations and provides an opportunity to rehearse safety behaviours. This can be useful for individuals during an acute crisis when their problem-solving capacity is compromised.

For the safety plan to be optimally effective, we need to understand an individual's story, to tease out what happened in the previous 24 hours. In particular we need to know the following:

- What factors were central to the suicidal thoughts and behaviour?
- What triggered the suicidal thoughts?
- Why did the suicide attempt happen on that occasion and not at another time?

It is also essential to check in with the person regularly to ensure that they are feeling okay. When completing the safety plan, it is also important to be flexible. Although the safety plan is numbered from Steps 1 to 6, it doesn't have to be completed in this set order. However, it is recommended that all six steps are completed. As it is structured around a conversation, be sensitive to the needs of the individual as they tell their story. They may find it difficult to share their private thoughts, so try not to stifle or constrain them, but, of course, it may be helpful to gently guide and prompt them. Utilising the widely-used person-centred interaction techniques from motivational interviewing may also be helpful, focusing on exploring and working with a person's values, goals, motivations and concerns.[15] The techniques or principles are usually summarised using the OARS acronym:

- **O**pen questions. When framing questions, try to avoid asking anything that is likely to yield a 'yes' or 'no' response, for example 'Are you suicidal?' Invite people to tell their story and find out what is important to them and what influenced their suicidal crisis.
- **A**ffirmations. Use verbal and non-verbal feedback to acknowledge effort and progress, no matter how small. Statements

and gestures that recognise and acknowledge strengths and behaviours that may lead to positive change will build the confidence that change is possible. They will also help to validate the person's experience. Many people who attempt suicide have had difficult upbringings and as a result their thoughts, feelings and behaviours may not have been validated so it is important to try to do so. Needless to say, these validations need to be genuine and authentic.

- **R**eflective listening. It is good practice to reflect back to the person what you understand by what they have told you and offer it back to them by 'paraphrasing' it. This gives them the opportunity to confirm your understanding and it also promotes engagement and trust.
- **S**ummaries. Similar to reflective listening, periodically offer summaries in the form of a concise overview of the key issues raised by the person. This is another opportunity to check understanding but it also provides focus following complex or lengthy discussions. It can also be helpful for transitioning to a new topic or direction.

## Step 1: Recognising warning signs

I get really, really short-tempered, fixated on the thought that I am such a bad person and I sleep a lot as I feel ashamed of how selfish I am.

This is the answer that Muhammad gave when he was asked what the warning signs were for his recent suicide attempt. He had attempted suicide before, and had thought a lot about the warning signs, therefore he was able to quickly come up with warning thoughts ('I am a bad person'), feelings ('I feel ashamed') and behaviours ('I sleep a lot').

When completing the safety plan, the warning signs that preceded a suicidal crisis should be explored collaboratively and recorded in the person's own words. Ask the person what sorts of things they notice, what thoughts and/or feelings they experience when they begin to feel suicidal. For some people, they have clear ideas about what the triggers are, but others, especially if there appears to have been little planning, may be unclear what the warning signs are. Always respond empathetically. It can be helpful to probe for specific thoughts, feelings or behaviours. Thinking of some examples can also help, such as:

- Thoughts: 'I am a complete waste of space'.
- Feelings: hopeless, trapped, overwhelmed, in despair, numb.
- Behaviours: risky behaviour, isolating self from others, self-neglect.

In the safety plan on page 195, there is only space for three warning signs, but this can be expanded, as some people generate multiple warning signs while others will only be able to think of one or two. In the SAFETEL study, warning signs included lack of sleep, nightmares, paranoia, racing thoughts, alcohol, restlessness, change in routine, sadness, overthinking, not being taken seriously, contact with ex-partner, negative thoughts and isolation.

It is also helpful to discuss that when the person experiences these warning signs then it might be a good time for them to seek out their safety plan. In such moments, they may want to work their way through it to keep themselves safe until the suicidal thoughts dissipate. People use their safety plan in different ways. Some people keep a folded-up copy in their wallet or handbag, others stick a copy to their fridge and others still keep a photograph of it on their phones. Some find it helpful to work their way through each step from Step 1 through to Step 6 when they feel a crisis escalating. Others skip steps or stop at a certain step if they begin to feel safe. Again, this is okay – the key thing is to use the safety plan in a way that works for the individual.

## Step 2: Identifying internal coping strategies

In Step 2, internal coping strategies are collaboratively explored with people. These are strategies an individual can use alone in order to cope better with suicidal thoughts/urges. Collectively, these would be things that are easily accessible regardless of location or time of day. To elicit these, you could ask what sorts of things they could use to distract themselves when they start to experience suicidal thoughts. These could be things that make them feel good, that they enjoy or that 'transport' them to a calmer place. Examples of coping strategies include:

- listening to favourite music
- drawing
- taking a relaxing bath
- playing video games
- watching TV
- walking the dog
- doing yoga
- going fishing

A key part of completing the safety plan is to explore the feasibility and safety of the coping strategies. This includes probing whether there are barriers to their use and what the likelihood is that the person will actually use the strategy during a crisis. Examining the barriers and facilitators of the coping strategies was probably the most important lesson that I took away from the training with Barbara and Greg. Take as an example Juliet, who was treated in hospital following a suicide attempt. She suggested 'going for a run' as one of her internal coping strategies. On the face of it, this was a reasonable suggestion. However, when she was asked what time of the day or night her suicidal thoughts tend to escalate, she said that this was usually late in the evening, not long before bedtime. So on reflection, going for a run late at night might not be the most sensible coping strategy, as it may not be physically safe. Another one of her suggestions was 'reading'. I, for one, cannot concentrate when I am feeling distressed, so again, don't forget to probe whether they will be able to use the strategy when in a crisis. Juliet confirmed, though, that wild horses cannot stop her from reading, so this was a good internal coping strategy for her to include in her safety plan. It can also be helpful to try to be as specific as possible. For example, if someone suggests reading or Netflix, it might be worth exploring what they might read or watch, perhaps gently steering them away from highly emotive or potentially depressing material.

In an exciting new study, using ecological momentary assessment, Barbara and colleagues found that people who were currently suicidal found distraction/positive activity-based strategies, such as keeping busy, thinking positively and doing something good for yourself, helpful in reducing the intensity of suicidal ideation in the short term.[16] People also said that they found mindfulness-oriented strategies like calming themselves and staying with feelings until they passed effective, but these didn't seem to reduce the suicidal intensity. Ecological momentary assessment is a technique in which people are asked in real time to tell us what they are doing and feeling in the moment, which they record on a mobile device.[17] It allows researchers to find out how changes in suicidal thinking over time are affected by other things, such as what they are doing to cope with their feelings.

## Step 3: Identifying people and social settings that can provide distraction

For this step, we are trying to identify people and social settings that can serve to distract individuals from their suicidal thoughts or urges. As the focus here is on distraction, there is no need to discuss feelings or emotions with the people included in this step. Once again, explore the feasibility, likelihood of use and any barriers. For anyone nominated, is this someone who they regularly chat with? Would they be happy to give them a call and/or consent to meet up with them? Through discussion, you are trying to clarify whether the people and social settings are suitable or not. If a gym is suggested, check what its opening hours are, so that it is open when the person is likely to need it to be. Clearly, bars and places where alcohol is served are best avoided.

Examples of people and social settings include:

- friends, family, acquaintances
- social settings such as coffee shops, parks, gyms, places of worship, museums, cinemas, libraries

Places to avoid include:

- bars, nightclubs
- environments where drugs are in use/available
- gambling settings (betting shops, casinos)

## Step 4: Contact chosen family/friends for support with suicidal thoughts/urges

Now the focus is on those people who the individual may find helpful to speak to when they are in a crisis. These are safe and trusted people who the individual will feel comfortable disclosing their suicidal thoughts to. As we go through the steps, we are moving away from monitoring risky signs and situations to more active responses to help to keep someone safe. This step is reached when the individual feels that the other steps have not or will not keep them safe. When working with the individual to complete this step, encourage them to think about whether this person will make them feel less upset. For example, it may not be wise to include an ex-partner who might be contributing to the individual's distress. The chosen family or friends should not be under the age of 18 and, as recommended for the previous two steps, think through the likelihood of use and any barriers to contacting people. Although not mandatory, asking if the person is willing to share a copy of their safety plan with the individuals listed in this step is good practice. At the very least, the contacts should agree to be included in the safety plan and know what might be expected of them. As many people who are suicidal are also socially isolated, or socially disconnected, be sensitive to the reality that they may not have someone to turn to in a time of need. The last thing we want to do is to highlight this to them, so it may not be possible to complete this section.

*Step 5: Contacting professionals for help*

This is a list of professionals and agencies that the individual can contact when a crisis is developing. These will be the organisations or professionals who the person can turn to if the previous steps are not sufficient to reduce their suicidal thoughts and urges and they are concerned for their safety. These will differ across countries but the key professionals and agencies will include: general practitioner, psychiatrist, community psychiatric nurse, crisis resolution and home treatment team, social worker, crisis helplines such as Samaritans, NHS 111 or the emergency services. As always, it is important to clarify the likelihood of and barriers to using such services during a suicidal crisis. For example, someone may find it helpful to save the telephone numbers of the professionals and agencies into their phone there and then, so they have them to hand in a crisis. It is useful to keep in mind that help-seeking is a behaviour so the principles of behavioural enaction are the same as for other behaviours. In other words, to increase the likelihood that we'll engage in them, especially during a crisis, it is critical that we think through the triggers, the barriers and the facilitators. In essence, like the VHS, the purpose of the safety plan is to increase the likelihood that help-seeking prevails over suicidal behaviour, when a suicidal crisis escalates.

*Step 6: Making the environment safe*

Whereas the previous steps of the safety plan are concerned with identifying warning signs and coping strategies, as well as listing people to contact in a crisis situation, the final step is focused on making the environment safe. Arguably, this is where we, as partners, parents or friends, could have the greatest impact, by helping our loved one to make their environment safe. In Step 6, we really need to work collaboratively with the individual to remove or restrict lethal means of suicide (e.g., large quantities of prescription drugs or other environmental triggers). Perhaps more than the other steps, the collaborative nature of this step is paramount, because it requires the individual to agree to make a change to their environment. The conversation may begin with a discussion of what they might use to hurt themselves when in a suicidal crisis and explore whether these things are available to them. It may also include a recognition that an important way to keep someone safe during a crisis is to plan ahead by removing or restricting access to the things that may cause them harm. Enquire about how we can make things safer and, specifically, try to agree a plan for doing so. The greater the specificity of the plan the more likely it is to be enacted.

Thinking back to implementation intentions, it is good to agree the how, the when and the where of keeping the environment safe. For example, if an individual is concerned that they'll take an overdose, they may agree to go home and immediately dispose of all toxic medications or agree to keep their medication in a locked box or ask someone else (e.g., a partner) to look after their medication. Clarify the plan, think through any barriers and, similar to the earlier barriers, try to problem-solve solutions.

Some people report that Step 6 can be the most difficult to complete, because there are practicalities and sensitivities about restricting access to lethal means. Indeed, speaking to colleagues in the US, there are particular sensitivities around restricting access to firearms. Ways around such difficulties have been to try to increase the distance between an individual and their firearm, or agreeing to the storage of ammunition separately from their firearm.[18] Another challenge with Step 6 is that it is extremely difficult to restrict access to areas of concern (e.g., bridges) or where the means of suicide are difficult to restrict (e.g., hanging). Despite being difficult, it is still possible to plan to stay away from such areas of concern (e.g., take a different route home from work, avoiding the risky area) or to restrict access to commonly available means of suicide (e.g., removing or locking away all ties or potential ligature material).

When the safety plan is complete, end the conversation by reviewing the safety plan and eliciting feedback from the individual to ensure everything that they wish to have included has been noted. Needless to say, the completion of a safety plan does not guarantee an individual's safety, but it certainly increases the odds that they will not act on their suicidal thoughts when they experience a suicidal crisis.

## The Safety Plan Pocket Card

Before moving on to longer-term interventions to keep people safe, Greg and Barbara have also developed a Safety Plan Pocket Card – the 5Rs of safety planning – which is an excellent aide-memoire for those delivering safety planning and which is reproduced verbatim below:[19]

| **Safety Plan Pocket Card** |
|---|
| <u>R</u>ationale of the safety plan<br>Explain:<br>• How suicidal crises come and go and identify warning signs (link to the individual's own experiences).<br>• How the safety plan helps to prevent acting on suicidal feelings.<br>• How the safety plan is a series of steps – go to the next step if the current step is not helpful (though it is not linear!). |
| <u>R</u>eact to the crisis to decrease suicide risk<br>Collaborate:<br>• To understand the reasons for each step.<br>• Brainstorm ideas for each coping strategy or resource.<br>• Be specific.<br>• Improve feasibility/remove barriers. |
| <u>R</u>emove access to lethal means<br>Work together to develop an action plan to:<br>• Limit access to preferred method or plan for suicide.<br>• Limit access to firearms. |
| <u>R</u>eview the safety plan to address concerns<br>Obtain feedback to assess:<br>• Helpfulness and likelihood of using safety plan.<br>• Where to keep the safety plan and when to use it.<br>• Was the safety plan helpful for preventing you from acting on suicidal thoughts? If not, why not?<br>• How can the safety plan be revised to be more helpful? |
| Gregory K. Brown and Barbara Stanley (2017) |

# 11

# Longer-Term Interventions

OVER THE PAST 25 years, there has been considerable growth in the number of RCTs of longer-term psychosocial interventions to reduce suicidal behaviour. As noted earlier, these longer-term interventions tend to involve a mental health professional who delivers a manualised treatment of some type of psychological therapy. If we take a look at the Cochrane Library of Systematic Reviews, despite this growth, the paucity of research is abundantly clear. The Cochrane Library is the gold standard in evidence reviews and is used to inform healthcare decision-making. In 2016, they published two reviews of the evidence for psychosocial interventions: one for the treatment of adults and the other for the treatment of children and adolescents.[1] Both of these reviews were led by Keith Hawton from the University of Oxford and they focused on all forms of suicidal behaviour including people who had self-harmed as well as those who had attempted suicide. Even though these reviews included brief contact interventions as well as longer-term interventions, there were only 55 trials covering 17,699 adults and 11 trials covering 1,126 children and adolescents.

The Cochrane reviews tend to apply very strict criteria for studies to be included, and, although the number of trials has continued to grow since these reviews were published, there still aren't enough. Indeed, there is nowhere near parity of esteem with physical health. For example, the charity MQ Mental Health Research has estimated that there is 25 times more money spent on research into cancer compared to mental health for each person affected.[2] And what's worse is that suicide prevention research only gets a fraction of this funding. Of course, I am not saying to stop funding research into cancer, I am just looking for some levelling up.

In this chapter, I describe the main psychosocial interventions that offer the most promise in terms of preventing suicidal behaviour. As I've noted elsewhere, although numerous scientific reviews show that such interventions reduce suicidal thoughts and behaviour, there is no evidence that they prevent suicide. This does not mean that they don't prevent suicide. Rather, that the sample sizes required to demonstrate a reduction in suicide are so large, that, for the most part, studies of the requisite scale just haven't been conducted.

As I take you through each therapy in turn, try to think of the active ingredients in each of the interventions and consider how they tap into the different components of the IMV model. You should see that there are many common features across the different approaches. Unfortunately, access to each of these therapies can be patchy and sadly waiting lists for treatment are also not uncommon. I'd recommend you contact your GP or family physician in the first instance as they will know what is available in your area and how to access treatment. Once again, though, if you think someone is at imminent risk of suicide, do not hesitate to contact the emergency services.

## Dialectical behaviour therapy (DBT)

Developed by the American psychologist Marsha Linehan from the University of Washington, DBT is a well-established treatment for suicidal behaviour and the condition borderline personality disorder (BPD). BPD is a mental health diagnosis characterised by emotional instability, disturbed thinking patterns, impulsive behaviour and intense but often unstable relationships with others. Linehan has been a towering presence in the psychological treatments field for decades. After dedicating her life to the treatment of mental health problems, Linehan, at the age of 68, revealed her own mental health fight for the first time. This included 26 months as an in-patient at the age of 17, followed by multiple suicide attempts and episodes of self-harm in the subsequent years. But over time and with a range of treatments she recovered. As she noted in an interview with the *New York Times* in 2011, she attributes her recovery to learning to accept herself as she was, together with the recognition that change was necessary.[3] Indeed, these dual attributions became the cornerstone of DBT, a cognitive behavioural therapy that combines a range of other concepts such as acceptance and mindfulness.

'Dialectical' comes from the word 'dialectic', meaning investigating contradictions and their solutions. In DBT, therefore, the aim is to resolve contradictory problems in people's lives by finding the balance between achieving acceptance and the need for change. One of its aims is to directly target suicidal behaviour or any behaviours that may interfere with treatment as well as other dangerous and destabilising behaviours. The latter may include some symptoms of BPD. DBT is an intensive intervention that combines weekly psychotherapy, group skills training and telephone support as well as consultations between therapists, usually delivered over 12 months. The findings from Linehan's seminal RCT of women with recent suicidal and non-suicidal behaviours were impressive. During the two years of the study, which included one year of treatment and one year of follow-up, those who received DBT were half as likely to attempt suicide and they were less likely to have been hospitalised for suicidal ideation.[4] More recently, there has been growing evidence that an adapted version of DBT – DBT-A – may be effective for adolescents with a history of repeated self-harming and suicidal behaviour.[5] In terms of adaptations, the duration of the intervention has been reduced for use with adolescents, being delivered over 19 weeks. However, like the adult version, DBT-A is also comprised of weekly sessions of individual therapy, family skills training, family therapy sessions and telephone coaching for individual therapists, as required. Overall, when the findings from different studies are synthesised, DBT for adults and adolescents seems to be effective in reducing the frequency of self-harm or suicidal behaviour rather than the proportion of people who self-harm or attempt suicide.

## Cognitive therapy (CT) and cognitive behavioural therapy (CBT)

Of all the psychosocial interventions targeting suicidal behaviour, most research effort has focused on CT and CBT. I am never quite clear what the difference between CT and CBT is because, from what I can see, they are often used interchangeably. In this section, I've stuck with using whichever term, CT or CBT, the authors of particular trials have used. CBT was developed by the

American psychiatrist and psychotherapist Aaron T. Beck in the sixties, as a new way of conceptualising and treating depression. His pioneering work was based on the cognitive model of depression.[6] The overarching premise of the cognitive model is that among individuals with depression, their information-processing system is operating dysfunctionally such that their view of themselves, the world and the future is distorted. This cognitive triad results in them believing that they're unlovable, that those around them think they're worthless and that things will only get worse in the future. According to Beck, these beliefs develop through a whole range of cognitive biases, such as negative automatic thoughts. These negative automatic thoughts are especially problematic when we are feeling stressed, as they are habitual and adversely affect how we feel and behave. They can lead us to become more self-critical, contribute to catastrophic thinking, when we believe that the worst is about to happen, and increase the likelihood that we see things in black or white, such that something is viewed as either only good or only bad. If you think back to the core elements of the IMV model, it is easy to see how these negative automatic thoughts (and other cognitive biases) may contribute to someone feeling defeated, humiliated, a burden and unbearably trapped.

Guided by the cognitive model, Beck developed CBT to challenge dysfunctional thoughts and behaviours, to improve emotion regulation and to develop problem-solving strategies, initially for depression. However, CBT has now been extended to a whole range of mental health conditions including suicidal behaviour.[7] Through a series of treatment phases, CBT helps the individual to reconceptualise their ways of thinking and behaving, and to acquire new skills to alleviate their distress and to navigate future challenges.

The definitive trial for the prevention of suicide attempts was led by Greg Brown and published in 2005. In collaboration with Beck, he found that adults who had attempted suicide were 50 per cent less likely to attempt suicide again over the next 18 months if they received CT designed specifically to prevent repeat suicide attempts than participants in the usual care group.[8] During the ten sessions of CT, the immediate thoughts, images and beliefs that seemed to be activated before a suicide attempt were identified, and cognitive and behavioural strategies were developed to help the individual cope with subsequent stressors and suicidal triggers. Other vulnerability factors, such as poor problem-solving, impulse control and social isolation, were also addressed as well as relapse prevention towards the end of therapy.

More recently, clinical psychologists David Rudd and Craig Bryan and colleagues have shown that a brief version of CBT was associated with a 60 per cent reduction in suicide attempts in a military sample, compared to those who received treatment as usual on its own.[9] Only time will tell whether this brief version of CBT is effective across other populations. Returning to the reviews that I mentioned earlier, the strongest evidence across different populations and different research groups is for CBT. Indeed, the Cochrane review concluded that there 'was a significant treatment effect for CBT-based psychotherapy' compared to usual treatment. However, it is not clear to what extent CBT is effective in reducing suicidal behaviour in children and adolescents. In large part, this uncertainty is because there are so few trials in young people. There is some evidence, however, that mentalisation-based treatment, a 12-month psychodynamic therapy, may be effective in reducing self-harm in adolescents.[10] This intervention, which includes both weekly individual sessions and monthly family therapy sessions, focuses on impulsivity and emotion regulation and aims to help the young person to better represent their feelings as well as those of others in difficult circumstances. In addition, another review by Dennis Ougrin from King's College, London and colleagues focused on therapeutic interventions for suicide attempts and self-harm in adolescents.[11] They concluded that there was evidence that therapeutic interventions worked, mostly driven by studies of DBT, CBT and mentalisation-based therapy.

In summary, what is evident across each of the different psychological interventions is that, although they may have different foci or guiding rationale, the same key processes emerge as targets for treatment, time and again. Indeed, these common elements – impulsivity, self-criticism, coping, imagery, problem-solving and self-worth – can all be mapped on to the IMV model.

## Collaborative Assessment and Management of Suicidality (CAMS)

CAMS was developed by David Jobes, a clinical psychologist from the Catholic University of America in Washington, DC, in the nineties.[12] CAMS focuses on identifying and targeting suicidal thoughts, urges and behaviours as *primary* targets for treatment as opposed to prioritising the underlying psychopathology. It is a therapeutic framework for the assessment and treatment of suicidal thoughts and behaviours. The guiding philosophy of CAMS is to stabilise vulnerable patients and to quickly engage them in the management of their own safety.[13] I have known Dave Jobes and his work for many years, we're good friends, but I remember being struck by a talk that he gave at the European Symposium on Suicide and Suicidal Behaviour in Glasgow in 2008. In that talk, he reiterated some of his thinking that underpinned the development of CAMS. Two points in particular stick in my mind from that talk. Although they relate directly to CAMS, they are applicable to all aspects of suicide prevention.

Firstly, to improve clinical care, Jobes has long argued that we need to move away from the reductionist view that sees suicide as a symptom or a by-product of mental illness. It takes more than the treatment of a mental illness to reduce suicidal thoughts and behaviours. He is clear in his view, and with which I concur, that the alleviation of the mental pain associated with suicidality takes more than medication. That is not to say that medication is not helpful in the treatment of mental illness. Rather, that the treatment of suicidality should be the central clinical target when working with patients who are suicidal. This, alongside the wider psychological suffering, should be core treatment targets.

Secondly, Jobes challenged the traditional 'Kraepelinian' approach (after the influential German psychiatrist Emil Kraepelin (1856–1926), who many regard as the founder of modern psychiatry) to the relationship between the patient and the clinician. Exponents of the latter approach tended to conceptualise the clinician as the expert and the patient or client as a passive respondent to their questions and recipient of their diagnoses. Jobes was keen to change the 'relational dynamic', away from a didactic approach to a collaboration, hence the inclusion of the word 'collaborative' in CAMS. Using the CAMS approach, the patient is an active collaborator in their care. Together with their clinician they work together to find a solution to their suffering. The clinician addresses suicidality directly, being empathic, acknowledging the patient's desire to die, but helping them to explore and agree alternatives. Not only is this a conceptual collaboration, but it is also literal, with the clinician sitting next to the patient during assessment and treatment planning, seeking to convey the message that they will work together to find a solution.

At the heart of CAMS is the Suicide Status Form (SSF), a clinical tool which is used throughout treatment, from assessment, to stabilisation planning and to treatment planning. At initial assessment, across three sections, the SSF is used to get a sense of how much psychological pain an individual is in. The circumstances associated with their distress, a comprehensive risk assessment and their own appraisal of their overall risk of suicide at that moment are conducted. The SSF is also structured to elicit reasons for living versus reasons for dying and to identify one thing that would help the person not to feel suicidal. The final section of the SSF is designed to facilitate the negotiation of the treatment plan. The treatment plan is organised around a series of problems for resolution, together with details of goals, objectives and interventions directed at achieving problem-resolution.

In terms of research evidence, to my knowledge, CAMS has been tested in five RCTs, with others in progress.[14] Across these studies, there is consistent evidence of CAMS being effective in reducing suicidal ideation, in community outpatients, in patients from specialised psychiatric care centres, in students and in soldiers. To date, though, each of the studies had relatively small sample sizes, rendering it more difficult to determine whether CAMS is effective in reducing suicidal behaviour.

## Attempted Suicide Short Intervention Program (ASSIP)

Despite the growing evidence base, a major challenge for longer-term treatment interventions is poor treatment consistency. Many patients feel that their clinician doesn't understand them or that their treatment isn't sufficiently patient-centred or collaborative (clearly CAMS and the other psychosocial interventions above are exceptions). To address these concerns, Konrad Michel and Anja Gysin-Maillart from the University of Bern in Switzerland developed ASSIP, with the clinical findings first published in 2016.[15] Its underpinning theoretical rationale is that suicide is a goal-directed action. According to this view, to understand suicide one needs to understand an individual's narrative, their beliefs, intentions and desires. Indeed, this view of suicide as a goal-directed action was an important influence on my own thinking when I was developing the IMV model. I still often quote Konrad Michel in talks, because he was the first person who I was aware of talking about suicide as a conscious behaviour and not merely a sign of illness and pathology. He has held this view for decades, and a long time before he co-developed ASSIP.

In terms of clinical influences, ASSIP prioritises the therapeutic alliance, which is the relationship between the clinician and the patient. It also draws heavily from clinical guidelines developed by an international working group, the Aeschi Group. This was a group of clinicians who first came together over 20 years ago because they were concerned about the quality of emergency assessment of patients following a suicide attempt. This working group also used to host a biannual conference in Aeschi, Switzerland to discuss new ways of thinking about therapeutic approaches to patients who are suicidal. As it happens, I had the good fortune to attend the second of these conferences in 2002.

I have vivid memories of the conference workshops in which Konrad would play back videos of patients telling their stories of suicidal thoughts and behaviours. We would dissect the conversations between the patient and their clinician, to identify best practice, to reflect and learn from these encounters. The six principles agreed by the Aeschi Working Group, to improve the therapeutic approach, are worth highlighting, and are clearly still relevant today:[16]

1. Work together with the patient to gain a shared understanding of their suicidality.
2. Be aware that most suicidal patients are in mental pain with little self-respect.
3. Be non-judgemental and supportive.
4. In a psychosocial assessment begin with the patient's own narrative.
5. The aim of the encounter is to engage the patient in a therapeutic relationship.
6. New models of suicidal behaviour are important to reach a shared understanding of the patient's suicidal state.

Although we still have some way to go, it is reassuring that most of the new psychosocial interventions, brief and longer-term, documented above are consistent with these principles. Even for a brief encounter such as safety planning to be effective, it must be collaborative, emerging from a shared understanding of suicidal distress. Indeed, it requires the speedy establishment of a supportive therapeutic relationship.

Returning to ASSIP, it is comprised of three clinical sessions that are followed up with semi-standardised letters over two years.[17] In the first session, the therapeutic relationship is established and the narrative interview detailing the patient's story that led to the suicide attempt is conducted. This interview is recorded, with the patient's consent, and then it is replayed in the second session. The aim is to gain a shared understanding of the suicidal crisis, focusing on the transition from suicidal thoughts to suicidal acts. The patient is also given a psychoeducation handout and asked to provide comments on it, as they recount and reflect upon their situation. In the third session, the handout is discussed, and warning signs and personalised safety strategies are agreed collaboratively and given to the patient alongside a list of crisis contact numbers and supports. Then, over a 24-month period, similar to the caring letters approach, the patients are sent a signed letter every 3 months in the first year and then every 6 months in the second year. These letters include a couple of personal sentences, but the bulk of the letter is a standard format, reminding them of the long-term risk of a suicidal crisis and the importance of safety strategies.

To date, there has only been one published RCT of ASSIP, but its findings are extremely encouraging. Across the two years of follow-up, there were only five suicide attempts and this is compared to forty-one in the usual treatment group.[18] That translates into an 83 per cent reduced risk of a suicide re-attempt. In addition, patients who received ASSIP spent 72 per cent fewer days in hospital during the follow-up period. Internationally, there are other research groups conducting trials of ASSIP in their countries, so let's hope that the findings are as positive.

## Digital interventions

Thus far, I've focused on the face-to-face delivery of interventions. However, this ignores the fact that most people who die by suicide are not in clinical care in the 12 months before death.[19] Therefore, they are unlikely to have benefited from the bespoke treatments described above. Moreover, as I have highlighted, the availability of face-to-face treatments tends to be patchy at best with waiting lists, so we need to consider alternative modes of treatment delivery. Add to this the reality that many of those who die by suicide may never have sought help in the past. As a result, digital interventions represent an important means of reaching those who do not seek help or who are currently excluded. These interventions can take different forms: some offer self-guided CBT for insomnia or depression, while others include mindfulness or safety planning.[20] Although digital interventions do not suit everyone, their widespread use is here to stay, especially in the post-COVID world. So what does the evidence say in terms of the suicide prevention properties of digital interventions?

In general, the evidence for digital interventions targeting suicidal thoughts and behaviours has lagged behind other online support for mental health problems such as depression and anxiety. However, colleagues in Australia have been spearheading efforts in developing and evaluating innovative suicide prevention digital interventions in recent years. For example, in 2019 Michelle Torok, a mental health researcher, together with Helen Christensen, chief scientist at the Black Dog Institute in Sydney, and colleagues published a review of self-guided psychological interventions for those at risk of suicide.[21] They found ten direct interventions, so called as they targeted suicidality, and six indirect interventions because they targeted depression rather than suicidality. Overall, they found that these interventions were associated with reduced suicidal ideation immediately following the end of intervention delivery.

They also found that it was the direct rather than the indirect interventions that were most effective. It seems, therefore, that apps or websites for the online treatment of depression are not likely to yield suicide prevention benefits on their own. This reinforces Dave Jobes' point that suicidality needs to be targeted directly in treatment irrespective of whether support is provided face-to-face or digitally.

It is also worth highlighting that the magnitude of the treatment effects for self-guided digital interventions are pretty similar to those for face-to-face treatments. However, there are lots of unanswered questions about the effectiveness of digital interventions. Similar to face-to-face treatments, it isn't clear whether they are equally effective for men versus women, for young people versus older adults, for people from different ethnic backgrounds or for those living in different parts of the world (e.g., high-income versus low- and middle-income countries). We also don't know what the active ingredients are, how long their protective effects last and, crucially, whether they actually reduce suicide attempts. The reality is that the science of digital interventions for suicide prevention is still in its infancy. But the outlook is positive. Although we still have much more to learn about their effectiveness, the evidence to date is promising.

In short, it is vital that evidence-based psychosocial interventions, digital or face-to-face, are available to those who need them. Too often those who present to emergency services in a suicidal crisis are discharged from hospital without a treatment plan or support in place. The evidence is clear – we need to do better, to ensure that continuity of care is prioritised. This may include safety planning, rapid referral, structured follow-up and support as a patient makes the transition from crisis into recovery.[22]

# Part 4

# Supporting People Who Are Vulnerable to Suicide or Bereaved by Suicide

As part of the national and international conversations around suicide prevention, people like me have been shouting from the rooftops 'If you are worried that a friend or family member may be suicidal, then please ask them directly.' In this final part, we hear from people who have asked the question – and how it has helped to save lives. However, asking the question about suicide is difficult, so I'll describe how to do this, and provide clear guidance/ tips, while building upon best practice. I hope to give you the confidence to ask about suicide – what I call the 'big S' question.

I also provide guidance for family members to help them to support their child or teenager who is having suicidal thoughts or who is self-harming. In addition, I'll address different ways to support a friend or colleague who is suicidal. Given that trauma is so common in people who are suicidal, we need to be more trauma-informed, being sensitive to the needs of family members, friends or colleagues who may be vulnerable as a result. In the final chapter, I explore the devastating impact of suicide on families, colleagues and friends, as well as on clinicians whose patients die by suicide.

# 12

# Asking People About Suicide

YOU MAY REMEMBER that there is no evidence that asking about suicide plants the idea in someone's mind, whereas it could be the start of a life-saving conversation (see page 52). Therefore, if you are concerned about someone's welfare, please ask them directly whether they are suicidal or not. It could get them the much-needed help and support that they require. In addition to the research evidence, I've also come across many real-life examples of people who have asked a friend or colleague whether they have been suicidal and this has been the catalyst for them getting help.

A few years ago, after a documentary I took part in was broadcast, a young person, Jack, emailed me to say that watching it had given him the confidence to ask a friend whether he was thinking of ending his life. The BBC programme in question was *Professor Green: Suicide and Me*, which was presented by the British rapper, who was on a personal journey to explore male suicide.[1] His interest was driven, in part, by trying to better understand his own father's suicide and he was shocked by the statistics that three quarters of all suicides in the UK are by men. Although he had rapped about the death of his father in his music, through songs such as his platinum-selling hit 'Read All About It', the documentary was the first time he had opened up to his close family about the circumstances around the death. It is an emotional film to watch, especially the parts with his nan, who looked after him for most of his early life.

As well as interviewing me to understand the psychology of suicide, Professor Green meets people directly affected by suicide or who have attempted suicide. One of those people was Ben, a former rugby player who had previously attempted suicide but who has since recovered and is doing well. It was this encounter that Jack found so helpful. Jack had 'never really thought that hard about why people killed themselves before' and it had made him think differently about suicide and mental health. Before watching the documentary, he just found suicide 'too scary' to think about and he believed that people who took their own lives 'were mentally ill and that there was nothing anyone could do to help them'. He had also thought that they were a 'different breed' from him until he saw Ben in the documentary. Ben reminded him of his own brother – they looked similar and had the same manner-isms. This helped Jack to recognise that people who are suicidal are just like anyone else. Then, a couple of weeks later, he was out having a few drinks with one of his mates, Abdul, who had just broken up with his girlfriend. It was clear that Abdul was pretty down, but they didn't tend to talk about emotions much, so initially Jack kept the conversation pretty light-hearted.

The break-up was the latest in a long list of difficult experi-ences that Abdul had gone through. That night, emboldened by watching the Professor Green documentary, Jack asked his friend whether he was suicidal. When he reflected on it, his efforts were clumsy because he just didn't know what to say, but they did the trick. Initially, Abdul seemed to be taken aback by the question, but then without saying anything he just started to cry. Jack learned afterwards that the tears were tears of relief because Abdul had never said the words 'I am exhausted and I just want to die' out loud before. So, as Jack stumbled over his words, it was like a weight had lifted for Abdul. He was also overcome with emotion because someone had realised that he wasn't well. He found it difficult to explain, but he felt safer; having shared his 'dark thoughts' with someone else for the first time, he felt a little more in control. The next day, Abdul contacted his GP and not long afterwards he saw a counsellor, who really helped him come to terms with the losses that he had experienced, including his relationship breakdown. He still struggled in the subsequent months, but Jack and Abdul had an agreement that if Abdul ever felt suicidal again he would contact Jack. And he did, a few weeks after their initial conversation. Abdul was feeling incredibly low and concerned that he couldn't keep himself safe. But just being able to chat openly with Jack was enough to get Abdul through his crisis until the next appointment with his counsellor.

Thankfully, stories like Jack's and Abdul's are becoming more and more common. Indeed, in Scotland, we recently launched a new suicide prevention public awareness campaign called 'United to Prevent Suicide'.[2] The aim of the campaign is to equip the general public with the knowledge, skills and confidence to talk about suicide and to be able to support someone to get the help that they need. It is aimed at all of us who might have a friend, acquaintance, colleague or family member who may be suicidal. We are building a social movement to prevent suicide, which is underpinned by the mantra that suicide prevention is everyone's business. And it is. The only way that we'll defeat the scourge of suicide is by all of us playing our own role in suicide prevention, no matter how small. That role can be simply raising a smile, reaching out to someone who is in distress or calling out mental health stigma whenever we see it.

The public awareness campaign 'Small Talk Saves Lives' launched by the mental health charity Samaritans a few years ago is another great example of how we can all play our part in suicide prevention.[3] Its key aim was to inform the general public that a little small talk could interrupt someone's suicidal thoughts and therefore help to save lives. It was a partnership with the British Transport Police, Network Rail and the wider rail industry in the UK to encourage people to strike up a conversation with someone at a train station or anywhere else for that matter. Their ask was simple: 'If you think somebody might need help, trust your instincts and strike up a conversation.' Crucially, though, when they were developing the campaign, they consulted people who had been suicidal in the past and were informed by research led by psychologist Lisa Marzano from Middlesex University.[4] Although it can be difficult to gauge the impact of such campaigns, within 15 days of its launch the multimedia campaign had reached more than 10 million people. Its reach was helped by endorsement from high-profile figures such as Stephen Fry and Lord Alan Sugar. The 'R U OK?' public awareness campaign is another great example from Australia of a social movement that is equipping thousands of Australians with what to say when someone says they're not okay. They provide tips and resources so that more people can have conversations that could potentially save a life.[5]

Scotland is recognised internationally as a country that has put suicide prevention front and centre of government policy over many years. This has been driven in large part by the fact that, for several decades, Scotland had the highest suicide rate out of the four nations of the UK. When I moved to Scotland in the late nineties, the suicide rate there was twice as high as that in England. And the suicide rate in the Highlands of Scotland was higher still. Things have improved considerably since then, with the suicide rates decreasing by 20 per cent in the intervening 10–15 years. Although it is not possible to know for certain what led to this reduction, since 2002 there has been a national strategy and action plan to prevent suicide.[6] Indeed, a key part of the strategy has been to highlight the importance of talking about suicide and asking for help. The action plan also led to thousands of people being equipped with suicide prevention intervention training, and thousands of people in distress receiving brief alcohol interventions. What is more, every local authority in Scotland developed their own local suicide prevention action plan tailored to the needs of their own communities. At the heart of the strategy was the idea that suicide prevention requires a public health approach, with local as well as national action, and that we can all play our part.

## Tips for Asking About Suicide

It can be difficult to ask questions about suicide, so I'll take you through some tips that I hope you find helpful. As part of the Scottish national suicide prevention response, NHS Health Scotland developed the 'Art of Conversation', a resource and campaign developed as a guide to talking, listening and reducing stigma around suicide.[7] It is an excellent resource, and perhaps one that Jack may have found useful when he was having his conversation about suicide with Abdul. The strapline for the resource says it all: 'Ask. Tell. Save Lives.' It tries to promote the idea that asking someone how they are feeling can make a positive difference. But the resource is so much more than its strapline. It includes information about myths, outlines key facts around suicide and highlights some of the warning signs that may indicate that someone might be suicidal. I have covered these warning signs elsewhere, but they are worth recapping here, all in one place, together with some others that I think are also important.

---

### WARNING SIGNS THAT SOMEONE MIGHT BE SUICIDAL

Someone may be thinking of suicide if:

- They are talking about being trapped, a burden on others and feeling hopeless about the future.
- They have experienced loss, rejection or other stressful life events and are struggling to cope.
- They are sorting out their life affairs, such as giving away prized possessions or getting their will in order.
- There is an unexplained improvement in mood. This may be because they have decided that suicide is the solution to their problems.
- There are marked changes in behaviours such as sleeping, eating, drinking, drug-taking or other risk-taking behaviours.
- They have a history of self-harm or have made a previous suicide attempt.
- They are acting or behaving unpredictably or out of character.

*Listen*

In my experience, a major barrier to asking about suicidal thoughts or self-harm is that people don't know what to say if a friend or family member replies with 'Yes, I am thinking of killing myself.' Of course, if someone says that they are thinking of killing themselves, it is understandable that this arouses fear and anxiety. You may be frightened that you'll say the wrong thing, that you will make matters worse or that you may not know what to do next. Some of this anxiety may be tied up in your desire to help them to solve their problems. But, sometimes, listening is enough, and it empowers them to seek help. Solving their problem is not your responsibility. This is something I am frequently guilty of. Instead of listening, I revert to problem-solving mode. As a result, in such situations I may miss crucial elements of what is being said. I am too busy trying to think of an answer for what to do next, to make things better. Although this is well-meaning, it may not be what a friend or family member wants or needs at that moment.

Never underestimate the power of listening; simply listening is so important, especially if we do so by also gently probing with open questions. This type of listening is called 'active listening', as the listener is concentrating on what the other person is saying, trying to make sense of what is being said and then responding. This allows the other person to decide what they feel comfortable disclosing and they remain in control of the conversation. Think back to the motivational interviewing techniques that I discussed on page 201 – this OARS technique should foster effective, supportive and active listening. The idea of control is also important to consider in this context as many people who are suicidal feel powerless and out of control.

Unsurprisingly therefore, even small instances of control can make a big difference and even lay the foundations for regaining control of events in one's life, as well as regaining control of one's emotions.

## Show compassion

In Scotland, we have developed the Distress Brief Intervention.[8] This is a multi-agency crisis response service for people in distress, spearheaded by the Scottish Government and involving a wide range of colleagues from the NHS, the education, social and voluntary sectors, and the police. I have had the privilege of leading the development of the intervention training for this service, alongside my colleagues Jack Melson and Karen Wetherall at the University of Glasgow. The reason for mentioning the Distress Brief Intervention here is because its mission is to provide connected compassionate support for people who are in crisis. To my mind, this is what we all should be trying to do when we are talking to people who are having thoughts of suicide: helping them to feel connected and supported compassionately.

Our conceptualisation of compassion in the Distress Brief Intervention is based on the work of the British clinical psychologist and author Paul Gilbert, who is one of the leading authorities on compassion and compassion-focused therapy globally. In his definition of compassion, he argues that compassion is more than simply being kind or caring.[9] Rather, it is also about having the courage to appreciate the causes of suffering in others and having the wisdom to know how to address these causes. Clearly, in an initial conversation, the focus is likely to be on being kind and caring. Nonetheless, it is really helpful to think about the courage and wisdom components as well. Fundamental to providing a compassionate response is being able to view things from the perspective of the person who is in distress. This requires empathy, which is the ability to both recognise and understand how someone feels.

We should also apply these same principles to ourselves, as self-compassion is crucial for our own well-being. Before I started my own personal therapy, I was incredibly self-critical and not very accepting of my own failings, and I spent too much time chastising myself. However, over the subsequent months and years of therapy, I have been able to nurture the courage and wisdom aspects of self-compassion and my mental health has definitely benefited. But you don't need to take my word for it. As I noted earlier, my colleague Seonaid Cleare reviewed the research literature and found that self-harm and suicidal ideation were less likely in people who reported higher levels of self-compassion.[10] So the next time you have a self-critical thought perhaps also think about something good that you have said or done that day.

## Build trust and collaboration

When trying to engage with someone who is suicidal, it is useful to remember that they may have a history of trauma or experienced adversity early in life. As we saw in Chapter 7, trauma experienced in childhood is particularly pernicious and it is an established risk factor for suicide. Moreover, this trauma may also impact upon their capacity to form relationships as adults. As a consequence, they may be distrustful of others, which may manifest itself as a reluctance to reach out or accept support when offered. This may explain, in part, the lack of engagement with clinical services and why people who have been suicidal are often described as being among the hardest to reach. I dislike the term 'hard to reach' because it is inaccurate and misleading. It isn't that these people are hard to reach. Rather, it is that we have failed to reach them. There are also often long waiting lists or other barriers to treatment engagement and too often people who are suicidal feel that the services are not tailored to their needs or that they have been let down by services.

In recognition of these engagement challenges, there has been a growing awareness of these barriers as well as the strategies to overcoming them. Indeed, Scotland was one of the first countries in the world to develop a knowledge and skills framework to ensure that the workforce in Scotland was aware of the impact of trauma and equipped to respond appropriately. The 'Transforming Psychological Trauma Framework', developed by NHS Education Scotland in partnership with the Scottish government and people with lived experience, aims to embed trauma-informed practice in all sectors of the workforce.[11] Moving forward, it is hoped that the needs of adults and children affected by trauma at any age will have their needs understood and met. The principles underpinning the framework are worth restating here as they are a useful shorthand guide when working with someone who has experienced trauma. Actually, I'd go one step further. They should be the foundation stones for any conversation with someone who needs help or support. The principles can be captured in five words:

1. Collaborate
2. Empower
3. Choice
4. Trust
5. Safety

As I tried to make clear in Part 3, the most effective interventions for suicide risk are all collaborative. The same principles hold when any of us are considering the needs of people who have experienced trauma, irrespective of whether we are a family member, friend or healthcare professional. When discussing potentially difficult topics, it is usually good to take a step back and try to see things from their perspective. Perhaps start by asking them what they need and try to work together to meet their needs. Help them to feel empowered, by working through options so that they are enabled to make decisions about what they need. Are there ways in which you can support them as they think through the pros and cons of what is on offer if you are trying to encourage them to consider getting support? If you are a healthcare professional, offer choices about their support. Of course there may be constraints, but for example, offering choice in the gender of the person offering the treatment or support may be particularly important if someone has been the victim of abuse. Try to build trust by being honest and clear throughout and, finally, ensure privacy and confidentiality. Needless to say, part of building trust will involve clearly communicating the limits of confidentiality, and that it may have to be broken if the person poses a risk to themselves or others.

Two final words come to mind when I think about how best to ask about suicide: be human!

# 13

# Supporting Those Who Are Suicidal

A HUGE CONCERN that we can all identify with is how we can best support a family member, friend or colleague who is suicidal or who may be self-harming. Of course, the nature of that support will depend on your relationship with the person or the family. In this chapter, drawing upon best practice, I'll highlight things to look out for as well as provide guidance to help you navigate these potentially difficult situations. This guidance builds upon the tips for asking people about suicide from the previous chapter as well as information from earlier chapters where I have tried to make sense of why people become suicidal in the first place. I'll start with a section on supporting families before moving on to supporting friends and colleagues.

## Supporting Families When a Young Person Is Having Suicidal Thoughts or Is Self-Harming

The first step in supporting the family of a young person who is suicidal or self-harming is to understand what they may be going through. Of course, the family you are trying to support could be your own or that of a friend's. However, I have written the following section about families in general, as I think this helps all of us to stand back and think about how we can best support others near and far.

Your family, or another family of a young person who is having suicidal thoughts or who is self-harming, will be trying to make sense of what is happening and come to terms with what this means for them and those closest to them. Feelings of failure, shame, guilt, shock and anger are common among parents and families of young people who are suicidal or who are self-harming. As parents, our most precious task is to keep our children safe from harm. And usually when we think about protecting our offspring, we are focused on protecting them against potential external harms, or trying our best to keep them physically healthy. The idea that our own child could harm themselves is an alien thought for most of us. But as I have noted elsewhere, the extent of adolescent self-harm serves as a sharp reminder. At least 1 in 10 adolescents will have self-harmed by the age of 16 and, of those, 1 in 5 will be girls, and they will have done so most likely in the preceding 12 months.[1] Even more still will express suicidal thoughts and some will be hospitalised following self-harm. Gender and sexual minority adolescents are also at increased risk of self-injurious thoughts and behaviours.[2]

The stigma and helplessness that families experience can be overwhelming, not knowing what to do or who to turn to. A few years ago, Anne Ferrey and Keith Hawton from the University of Oxford published an interview-based study of parents whose son or daughter had self-harmed.[3] The findings were moving and highlighted the urgency around supporting families through these difficult times. Parents talked about the immediate impact of discovering that their child had been self-harming; the shock, the disbelief as well as the ongoing impact on their own mental health. Some of the parents reported becoming depressed, being emotionally exhausted, becoming hyper-vigilant and overprotective. The impact on siblings was also wide-ranging, with some parents reporting that their other children were resentful and angry, with others saying that siblings were supportive. There were also reports of siblings feeling responsible for their brother's or sister's self-harm and others felt the stigma of having a sibling who self-harmed. All in all, these interviews highlighted the pervasive and painful impact on families of having a child who self-harms or who is suicidal. Unsurprisingly, the strain on the family unit also exposes any pre-existing tensions or cracks in relationships, which can further contribute to the emotional load on all members of the family. These are the sorts of issues, therefore, that you may want to hold in mind when you are trying to support a family where a young person is self-harming or is suicidal. If you are a parent in this situation, it is important to recognise that you will be experiencing many different, often conflicting, emotions. As mentioned elsewhere, try not to be hard on yourself and avail yourself of the support offered by family and friends, as well as that from professionals.

Another overarching theme that emerged from these interviews was a deep sense of isolation experienced by many of the parents and the value of and need for social support. Some of the parents found the informal support offered by friends to be helpful, but for others they felt that they would have benefited from support groups. Unfortunately, to my knowledge, there are very few such support groups available. It doesn't matter whether you live in Glasgow, Beijing or New York, the options for support are limited. Overall, these research findings resonate with my experience of meeting numerous families over the years who have had a child who has self-harmed or attempted suicide. Once they have overcome the initial shock, they have so many questions swirling around in their head that need answers: How can I keep my child safe? Who can I turn to for support? How could I have failed my child? What will others think of me and my family? How can I get help while maintaining my child's privacy? The reality is that there are no easy answers to these questions, but they underpin the vast unmet need of families trying to cope with a child who is suicidal or self-harming. These are some of the key issues that this chapter seeks to address.

There are so many tensions at play when families are trying to cope with such difficult circumstances. I remember these tensions coming up in a conversation I had with a family whom I met a few years ago. I had just given a public lecture on adolescent suicide and self-harm and the formal question and answer session had finished, but there was a couple who had waited for me, after everyone else had left. I had already spotted them during the evening, as the father had become emotional during one part of my talk and, when I caught his eye, he nodded as if to say, 'I am okay, it's fine.' So I was pleased that they had stayed behind as it gave me the opportunity to check in with him.

At that time, they were still living through what the father described as 'an utter nightmare'. Their son Arron, 15, had struggled with friendships since primary school. He had become a 'loner' and his self-esteem had hit 'rock bottom'. Arron just kept thinking that no one liked him, mainly because he was a bit different from his peers. Even now, he had no one he could call a best friend. When puberty hit, things got much worse and he also struggled with his sexuality. He had a really 'dark period' not long after his thirteenth birthday, but his parents thought things were better more recently. He seemed content with his own company, spending a lot of his free time on his PlayStation. This didn't seem to be that different from many other adolescents, so they didn't think much of it. But then, about two months before I met them, Arron's sleep became really disrupted and then, completely out of the blue, one night they found him unconscious after taking an overdose that resulted in hospitalisation. Despite the medical severity, Arron was extremely fortunate as there was no residual medical damage and he was discharged two days later. But the family was floored. His parents felt so guilty, so ashamed that they had failed him and petrified that he would do it again. Arron said the overdose was impulsive, he couldn't explain why he had done it, he was just 'overwhelmed'. Like so many of the parents interviewed in Anne Ferrey's study, they were in shock. It felt like an assault on them as parents; by harming himself, it felt like their son was attacking them. Of course he wasn't, but they couldn't help but feel anger and resentment towards their son. These are key emotional and understandable reactions to look out for when supporting families.

Arron's parents just couldn't process how things had escalated so quickly or how they hadn't seen it coming. When they reflected on what happened, they had been anxious about their son in the weeks beforehand because he had been a little unpredictable and aggressive. But they just never thought he'd take an overdose. They had put his agitation down to the storms of adolescence, him trying to make sense of his sexual identity and his disturbed sleep. They had come to my talk in the hope that it would help them understand what had happened. They knew already that I couldn't give them specific answers, but they were keen to share their story and wanted to know what else they could do to keep their son safe. I explained that I wasn't a clinician. I encouraged them to see their son's GP again and to ensure that there was a safety plan in place. They felt helpless and let down by the NHS. Even though their son had taken an overdose, as he had denied any suicidal intent, he wasn't deemed as high-risk. The family was told that there was a long waiting list for treatment. In their eyes, when their son needed the safety net of the NHS around him, it just fell away, leaving him and the family to deal with this situation with no support. I hope this book can help parents who are going through such awful ordeals, by providing some hope and advice as they struggle to keep their child safe and well.

Sadly, their experience is not uncommon; in the UK, and in many countries, the waiting lists for treatment for child and adolescent mental health are unacceptably high. This is not the fault of dedicated frontline staff, who, in my experience, are as frustrated as I am by these delays to treatment. We often hear politicians talk about the importance of ensuring parity of esteem between mental and physical illness, for example, in terms of waiting times to treatment. Although some progress has been made in this regard in recent years, sadly this remains largely an aspiration rather than a reality. Arron's family's experience of being lost at sea, being uncertain about what to do to best support and protect their child, mirrors that of countless others. More needs to be done to deliver timely support for young people and their families. Always remember that if you are concerned that a young person is at imminent risk of suicide, without hesitation contact the emergency services.

We also need to think about managing the risk of self-harm and suicidal behaviour in schools. Although there are challenges in doing so, a large European study led by Danuta

Wasserman from the Karolinska Institute in Sweden found that a structured programme called Youth Aware of Mental Health (YAM) is effective in reducing suicide attempts and suicidal ideation in adolescents.[4] This is a peer support programme where young people are encouraged to talk about their mental health and to discuss issues that are important to them. Even if it is not possible to implement the programme in full, schools should endeavour to adhere to its principles by encouraging safe spaces for young people to role-play and discuss their mental health and well-being.

In the last few years, some excellent online resources have been developed to help parents and carers cope with a child's self-harm. For example, building on the interviews with families, Anne Ferrey and Keith Hawton produced an online resource called 'Coping with self-harm: A guide for parents and carers'.[5] It starts with an explanation of what self-harm is and the reasons for self-harm and it emphasises why it is important to tackle self-harm early on. In the next section I have drawn upon their guidance to outline practical things that parents or carers can do to cope with self-harm.

## Communication, communication, communication!

Good communication is the start, the middle and the end of supporting your child. It is absolutely vital to coping with self-harm. However, sometimes it is difficult to do so effectively, especially if you are in shock, you are angry with your child or they are angry with you. As we saw above, Arron's parents were so conflicted – they loved him but were also angry and petrified. So, what can be done to make communication more effective? The 'Coping with self-harm' resource offers some helpful tips, which I summarise in the next few paragraphs together with some of my own thoughts. However, in acknowledgement of the challenges in coping with a child's self-harm, I have deliberately framed many of the tips as things you should try. This recognises that coping with self-harm is difficult, so try not to be self-critical when you inevitably become impatient, frightened or frustrated. Such responses are understandable.

Try to initiate a conversation, but do so gently, and, if your child is willing, ease into bringing up self-harm. To reduce the intensity, perhaps arrange to do another activity – go for a walk or a drive – and then have the conversation. Arron's parents lived by the seaside, and they went for a walk on the beach a few days after his overdose to talk about what happened. A young person may try to deny the self-harm at first or they may not know what to say. Lots of emotions are likely to be at play. They may feel ashamed or embarrassed or angry, or all three at once. If they do deny that they have self-harmed, that's okay, perhaps try again later. But always give them a way out when you ask them any difficult questions. If they feel boxed in or cornered, you are unlikely to get very far and it could lead to resentment. It could also add to feelings of being trapped. As far as possible, give them an opportunity to try to explain and make it clear that you'll listen to them. Try to be non-judgemental and tell them that you love them and that you'll always love them, no matter what they say. Tell them that the act of self-harm doesn't alter your love for them.

Try not to be offended if they don't want to speak to you. Suggest to them that they may wish to talk to someone else – this could be a professional like a GP or another health professional. Also consider that they may not want to talk face-to-face, but they might be open to a text message, WhatsApp message or email. When asking questions about why they self-harmed, try to frame them as 'What happened to you?', and avoid negatively loaded statements such as 'What's wrong with you?'

Your child may be struggling to understand why they are feeling the way they do, especially if they are negotiating adolescence and trying to work out who they are. They may also be 'trying out' different identities. As much as possible, try to convey validation, empathy and compassion to your child. It is so important to validate how they are feeling. Even if you cannot understand why they feel the way they do, it is a reality for the young person. Try not to minimise how they feel. You should also show empathy by telling them that you understand how they feel and display compassion by expressing concern for their suffering and that you want to help them to reduce their suffering. Even if they may look fine to you, they are evidently struggling inside and always try to remember that they are the experts in how they feel. Some parents find this difficult to accept, thinking that they know best.

Once communication is established, try to help them identify the triggers to their self-harm. Using the VHS (page 148) or a safety plan (page 195) – if they have one – may be useful for this, as well as structuring thinking around how to respond differently the next time they encounter these triggers. In the same way as I suggested for safety planning, try to work together to think about potential alternatives to self-harm (see the next page).

## Identify coping strategies

Try not to define your child by their self-harm. Remind them of their strengths and that they are not a failure and that their struggles will pass. For a young person, it can be particularly difficult to see beyond their current crisis. Reassure them that things will get better in the future and that even if they don't have an answer now about what might help, they can keep working at it and they may find it helpful to ask their doctor.

Thinking beyond the current episode of self-harm, try to consider alternatives. Help your child think about other ways to cope with their feelings and emotions. These alternatives could be distraction techniques, such as watching a movie or listening to music, or they could be soothing, like having a bath or drawing or doing something else creative. Thinking about different ways of releasing emotions can also be helpful. What works for one young person may not work for another. However, holding an ice cube tight until it melts or pinging an elastic band around the wrist may offer some release. Some young people say that doing sports or exercise, drawing on the skin with a pen or punching something soft like a pillow can also be effective stress-reduction activities.

## Who to tell?

Knowing who else to tell is tricky. It is important to think about their reactions. Will they be frightened? Will they under-stand? These decisions are always a fine balance between the need for privacy and the need for support. Similarly, talk through with your child whether you tell other family mem-bers such as siblings. Again, there is no right or wrong answer, and it is a case of thinking through the benefits and harms of secrecy versus telling them. The other siblings may also need support to manage their own emotions because even if the self-harm is not disclosed, they may have sensed that something isn't quite right.

Who to tell may also include the digital world. The young person may have already shared their experiences online or they may be considering doing so. Jo Robinson and her colleagues from the Centre for Youth Mental Health in Melbourne, Australia have co-developed #chatsafe with youth networks, an incredibly helpful young person's guide for communicating safely online about suicide and self-harm.[6] These resources have been modified for use in different countries and provide practical tools and support around posting online. Specifically, #chatsafe describes things to reflect upon when a young person wants to share their own thoughts and feelings online. These include reminders that posts can go viral and that it can be difficult to delete posts once they are posted, as well as useful tips on monitoring a post after it has been posted. They also offer some practical tips on self-care for a young person. #chatsafe also provides guidelines about memorial websites in the tragic event of the suicide death of a young person.

## The role of the GP

The role of the GP in managing self-harm or suicide risk should not be underestimated; indeed, they are usually the gatekeepers of the care that we receive. Whereas most people who die by suicide have not been in touch with mental health services in the year before death, between at least 60 and 80 per cent of people under the age of 35 have seen their GP within 12 months of their suicide.[7] In addition, more than half of the young people who self-harm have also been in touch with their GP in the preceding six months.[8] There is huge potential for GPs to identify and manage suicide risk not just in young people but in people across the whole of the lifespan.

Of course there are many challenges for GPs. First, their consultation times are often limited to less than ten minutes so it can be difficult to conduct a detailed psychosocial assessment in this time. Second, although the majority of people who die by suicide present to their GP or primary care practice nurse in the 12 months before death, they do not always disclose whether they are suicidal or not. To address the latter, I'd urge every GP to directly ask every patient who they are concerned about whether they have thoughts of suicide and, if yes, whether they have a plan and to respond accordingly.

Although the following section has been written with a GP in mind, if you are a parent of someone who is suicidal or self-harming, it should provide you with some guidance about what to expect from a GP. The key principle here is for the GP to engage the person in a conversation and not to rely upon risk assessment scales or tools. By talking to the patient, the GP can bring together information about their past and integrate this with the present life circumstances, to build up a picture of the patient's needs as well as their risks. Consistent with the National Institute for Health and Care Excellence (NICE) guidance on the management of self-harm, just to reiterate, a GP should not rely solely on clinical risk tools and scales to ascertain risk of suicide. They just don't work. As my good friend and colleague, Nav Kapur, the head of research at the UK's National Confidential Inquiry into Suicide and Safety in Mental Health at the University of Manchester, has been saying for years, there is no evidence that such tools or scales predict suicide. Indeed, their use can provide a false sense of reassurance. In short, clinical care should never be decided solely on the basis of insights from such tools.[9] Of course, the use of such tools may be helpful as part of a more holistic psychosocial assessment or as a means of structuring a discussion around suicide risk. Indeed, they can provide valuable information that the GP as well as the family can use to help support the young person.

Instead of second-guessing what young people who self-harm or who are suicidal want from their GP, Jo Robinson, India Bellairs-Walsh and colleagues asked a group of young people in Australia for their views.[10] Once again, if you are a parent or a GP these insights are invaluable as they will help you to understand precisely what a young person wants and needs when they go to see their GP. These discussions gave rise to five interrelated themes.

The first theme revolved around wanting a collaborative dialogue. I am beginning to sound like a broken record now, but collaboration is at the heart of everything we need to do to help to manage self-harm or prevent suicide. The days of paternalistic views, such as the health professional knows best about someone else's mental health, are gone. Also, the young people wanted the GP to be proactive, to ask questions about their mental health as well as their physical health. Some of the young people said that the GP just didn't fully explore their suicidality and that this was a missed opportunity to help. We need to learn from these findings. The collaborative dialogue should also extend to treatment options, including the benefits and risks of different decisions. According to the young people, this approach is important to promote patient autonomy and informed decision-making. If you are a parent, this may be something to discuss with the GP together with your child.

The second theme – fearing a loss of privacy when disclosing risk – acted as a barrier to some of the young people disclosing personal details about their mental health and suicidal thoughts. This is something for both parents and the GP to consider when thinking about what the young person may be worried about. In the Australian study, young people were concerned about what information would be recorded in their medical records and where this information may go, especially as health records are becoming increasingly digitalised. This theme highlights the need for transparency and clarity from the GP about what will happen with a patient's personal information and to whom it will be disclosed.

The third theme focused on the labels that GPs used; for example, some of the young people didn't like the term 'at risk'. It was seen as negative and intimidating and they encouraged GPs to think about using more positive language perhaps with a focus on well-being rather than risk. They also wanted more focus on their symptoms and experiences, seeing them as a whole person, rather than being reduced to diagnoses. There was also push-back on the traditional medical approach of someone being either well or sick, which they found problematic and in some cases invalidating. This is useful advice for all of us to remember – to look beyond any labels or diagnoses, and try to see the world and the young person's struggles through their eyes.

Related to the previous theme, the importance of GPs' attitudes was emphasised in the fourth theme. Understandably, if the GP comes across as indifferent or conveying an impersonal attitude, then young people will be put off from seeing their GP and it will definitely act as a barrier to disclosing mental health problems. Needless to say, the substance of this theme applies equally to everyone who is supporting a young person; from family members to friends and from teachers to health and social care professionals. Young people also do not appreciate a GP–patient interaction that is formulaic and 'tick-box' focused. Active listening, good eye contact and an engaging posture were also raised by the young people as important when they are discussing their suicidality or self-harm. We should all keep in mind that the young person will feel vulnerable when self-disclosing such private information, so we should avoid being judgemental or dismissive, or minimising their concerns.

The final theme to emerge was that the young people recognised how important GPs are in the provision of practical support. They were seen as such a valuable resource at a time of crisis and some felt it important that they were offered follow-up support. The latter is not surprising because too many young people who self-harm or who are suicidal don't feel valued, so a GP – or other professional – showing interest in their well-being over time can be very powerful.

## Look after yourself

As Anne Ferrey and Keith Hawton's research demonstrated, the emotional impact on parents and carers is considerable. So, the final *try* in this section is: please try to remember to look after your own well-being if you are a parent or carer. Of course, in the midst of a crisis, this can be difficult to do, but it is crucial. Take time for yourself. If you don't attend to your own needs you will not be in a position to look after the needs of your children.

> If you feel that the safety of your child is at risk, always seek professional help, from your GP or a mental health professional, or contact a helpline. And don't hesitate to contact the emergency services if you think your child's life is in immediate danger. I have included a list of resources, including places to go for help, on page 277.

## Supporting a Friend or Colleague Who Is Suicidal

Having lost two friends who were also colleagues to suicide, I don't know if I am the best person to comment on supporting a friend or colleague who is suicidal. Except, I've spent a lot of time since my friend Clare died reflecting on my own experiences. On several occasions, Clare and I discussed her suicidal thoughts and I have a vivid recollection of the final time we had an in-depth conversation about the pain she was experiencing. She did feel trapped and she was mentally exhausted. That conversation ended with tears, a big hug, with my then-toddler daughter interrupting us and jumping all over Clare. They adored each other and, as Clare found mornings difficult, when she came to visit she would get up early with my daughter while the rest of us slept. It was a special bond for both of them.

That last discussion about mental pain was some months before Clare's death, but I have thought often about what I could have done differently. Of course, I cannot alter the past, but I keep coming back to the thought that I wasn't direct enough. Although we talked about her feeling hopeless, as far as I can remember, we never discussed whether she might ever act on her thoughts. I have racked my brain for an answer as to why we didn't. Was it that I just thought that there was no way that she would act on her thoughts, so I didn't ask? Or was I just too frightened to ask in case she said yes? Or did Clare not want to go there, and I picked up on this, implicitly? The honest answer is that I just don't know why I didn't ask. And that's a regret that I still live with. I think I could have supported Clare more. In my replaying of history, I would have taken her mental pain more seriously, but I didn't. So my advice is, if you are supporting someone who is expressing suicidal thoughts, always ask them directly 'Have you thought about acting on your thoughts?' If the answer is yes, then explore help-seeking and safety planning with them and, as I've said before, if you are concerned that they are not safe, urge them to get in touch with a professional. And if they are reluctant, ask if you can do it for them. Ultimately, though, if they don't agree and you think they are at imminent risk of suicide, you may have to contact the emergency services.

It can be difficult to spot if someone is suicidal because many people will try to keep their feelings a secret and appear as if nothing is wrong. But keep an eye and an ear out for warning signs that they are struggling to cope. I outlined these on page 234, but they are worth restating again. Warning signs may include feelings of being trapped or being hopeless. Being agitated, engaging in risky behaviours, reports of loneliness and thinking they are a burden on others would be red flags worth exploring. I have mentioned loneliness a few times without saying something more concrete about the evidence linking it to suicide risk. My colleague Heather McClelland addressed this very issue in a review we conducted, and the findings were clear.[11] Loneliness predicts suicidal thoughts and behaviour over time and the association is likely explained by increased depression in those who are lonely. However, we couldn't say anything about the relationship between loneliness and suicide itself as we couldn't find any studies that had investigated this relationship over time.

If you go back and look at the IMV model (page 102), you'll find more potential warning signs there. Without question, if a friend or colleague says that they're suicidal, always take it seriously. As I said at the start of the book, about 40 per cent of people who die by suicide will have told someone beforehand that they're suicidal. Telling someone else that they are suicidal is a good thing because it suggests that they're reaching out for help. Also, it is a brave thing to do, as they may have been reluctant to disclose their feelings. They may be anxious not knowing how you will react. So, if a friend or colleague does say they're suicidal, try not to be judgemental. Try not to react with shock, dismay or disbelief. Compassion and empathy are needed, otherwise they may close down again emotionally.

# 14

# Surviving the Aftermath of Suicide

THE IMPACT OF bereavement by suicide on those affected is vast. As I wrote at the start of Part 1, it is likely that as many as 135 people knew the person who died. In the largest study of its kind, Sharon McDonnell from Suicide Bereavement UK led a survey of over 7,150 people in the UK who had been bereaved by suicide.[1] She asked them about the impact of suicide as well as their access to support services. The findings were published as a report entitled 'From Grief to Hope: The collective voice of those bereaved or affected by suicide' in 2020. Four out of five people who responded said that the death had a major or moderate impact on their lives. More than one third reported mental health problems and 38 per cent had thought about ending their lives. For too long the voices of people bereaved by suicide have not been heard and they have not been adequately supported. Thankfully this is changing, but there is still a long road ahead.

In 2017 the British Radio DJ and TV presenter Zoe Ball lost her partner Billy to suicide. I remember reading about her loss in the national media. She was so overwhelmed with grief and, like so many people bereaved by suicide, she struggled with the question 'Why?'; why could she not have saved the person she loved? With time she has said that she has come to accept that she couldn't have done anything to save him. She has taken a little comfort in the knowledge that Billy's pain has ended. Her loss spurred Ball on to embark on a gruelling 350-mile Sport Relief fundraising bike ride to raise awareness about mental health and to shine a light on the scale of male suicide and the extensive unmet need of men in emotional distress. Her heroic efforts were certainly not in vain as she raised over £1 million for mental health organisations across the UK.

On World Suicide Prevention Day in 2019, nine months after losing her partner Wayne to suicide, Amy Irons, the Scottish sports presenter, talked about the unbearable and horrendous pain that she had gone through as she battled with her own mental health. Her post on Twitter at the time was powerful. It highlighted her pain as well as urging people to reach out, ending with a message of hope:[2]

Losing Wayne through suicide left me questioning life myself. If I can say anything this #WorldSuicidePreventionDay it would be, please speak to people, don't be ashamed or hide how you feel, you aren't alone. And above all please hold out for the better days, I'm so glad I did.

Her Twitter post is a brief intervention in itself. It has some of the characteristics of the caring letters that I described on page 189, offering hope that things can get better. A few weeks later, I met Amy when I was doing a BBC Scotland interview about the publication of the latest suicide statistics in Scotland. I was struck by her passion around mental health promotion, especially her message for men to reach out for help. Without doubt her post will have helped innumerable people, both those who struggle daily to stay alive and those who have been bereaved by suicide. Indeed, the thread of comments below her post was a testament to the help and support that her message provided.

Sadly though, a few months later, I heard Amy on BBC Radio Scotland. But she wasn't talking about sport. In an emotional broadcast, she was talking about online trolling. She had been the victim of an anonymous malicious Instagram account, the author of which messaged her to ask, 'Was it your fault that your boyfriend took his life?' This is utterly despicable and completely unacceptable, but there was little she could do. Although most people who lose a loved one to suicide are not in the public eye, this post highlights a wider issue, which extends beyond online trolling. I have lost count of the number of times that a bereaved husband, wife, partner or other family member has disclosed their unbearable pain because they think that the suicide of their loved one *was* their fault. So, it is easy to see how such distasteful messages can be so overwhelming because for many people who are bereaved they are blaming themselves already. I touched on this issue earlier in the book: the pain they are already feeling is further exacerbated by thoughts that perhaps others are also blaming them for the death of a loved one.

Meet Andy, whose story illustrates the guilt and the blame that so many people bereaved by suicide report, especially in the early days following the death of a loved one. Andy and Michael, both in their late twenties, had known each other for several years. They had only been in a relationship for nine months and living together for about four before Michael's death, which came completely out of the blue. They both shared a pretty extensive history of mental health problems since their late teens. As Andy told me one afternoon over the phone, they used to joke that it was him who was more likely to kill himself and definitely not Michael. Andy had spent much of his early twenties with his arms in bandages, as a result of repeated self-harm. Conversely, although Michael had been on medication for ADHD and anxiety since he was 18, to Andy's knowledge, he had never self-harmed or attempted suicide. In the run-up to his death, Michael had been grappling with his past. After being brought up in the care system, he had recently made contact with his birth mother. This reunion had really unsettled Michael. It wasn't what he had hoped for, and it seemed to coincide with him starting to drink heavily. Andy wasn't a big drinker, so Michael's drinking had led to quite a few arguments. From what Andy could tell, he just seemed to be angry with the world. It was as if meeting his mother had unleashed a lifetime of hidden pain that had been dormant for years. The last time that Andy saw Michael alive, they had a major argument, which resulted in Michael storming out, in tears. This had happened before so Andy wasn't unduly concerned. He went to bed, expecting to find Michael beside him when he awoke the next morning.

But Michael never did come back. He was reported missing the next day and it took another three days for his body to be found, in some waste ground not that far from where they lived. When I spoke to Andy, it was coming up to the 12-month anniversary of Michael's death. He told me how he had many more good days than bad now, which he viewed as good progress. But when the bad days descended they were just as awful as they had been when Michael first died. Even though he keeps telling himself that he couldn't have done anything differently, on those dark days his mind is continually drawn back to that final argument, and to the painful 'Why?' questions that I talked about earlier. Why did he not just bite his tongue instead of having the argument that night? Why wasn't he more sensitive to Michael's needs? Why did he not phone Michael after he left the flat? Of course, on the good days, he has different answers to these questions: 'An argument takes two people, not one. He had been incredibly supportive of what Michael was going through, but it just wasn't enough. Michael could have called him; why was it always up to him to make the first conciliatory move after they had an argument?'

These are questions that we have all grappled with in relationships, but thankfully, for most of us, we don't have to revisit the answers after someone close to us has taken their life. When Andy feels his darkest, he becomes obsessed with the thought that other people blame him for Michael's death. He finds this so unbearable because part of him believes that he was to blame and he is convinced that he overheard a conversation between some of Michael's work colleagues saying that he was responsible for Michael's suicide. But when we discussed this further, there didn't seem to be any evidence that they had said what he had thought.

In the first six months after his loss, Andy didn't want to talk to anyone outside of his immediate family circle about his loss, least of all 'expose himself to a well-meaning support group'. Reluctantly, though, on the advice of his GP and nudges from a couple of friends, he started attending a Survivors of Bereavement by Suicide (SOBS) group. He has found this incredibly helpful. SOBS is a national organisation in the UK that provides support for anyone over the age of 18 who has been bereaved by suicide. This has allowed him to come to terms with his guilt and to accept that he wasn't responsible for Michael's death. It has also helped him with the isolation and the stigma that he felt so keenly and now he is such a strong advocate of such groups. But for every person I know who has found such groups helpful, I can think of others who chose not to go down this path. For me, the important element is that people who are bereaved should have choice. Such support should be available to anyone who needs it. Unfortunately, this just isn't the case. Bereavement support tends to be delivered by charities, which exist largely from the proceeds of fundraising. They are often not able to meet the demand. It is a disgrace that dedicated suicide bereavement support is not routinely available across the country. Indeed, two of the recommendations from the Suicide Bereavement UK report relate to this. The first recommendation calls for the implementation of national minimum standards in bereavement support services and the other appeals for the establishment of a national online resource for those bereaved or affected by suicide.

## Supporting Those Who Have Been Bereaved By Suicide

Everyone's experience of grief following a suicide death is unique, but there are some thoughts, feelings and emotions, such as guilt, anger and hopelessness, that are common. And there are many excellent books, often written by or with input from people who have been bereaved by suicide, that can be really helpful.[3] But as a husband who lost his wife told me recently, these books on suicide bereavement are all well and good, but in the early days of bereavement, he just wasn't able to concentrate for long enough to read them. So, he usually resorted to searching the Internet, often getting lost down a virtual rabbit hole of self-help websites. On one of those forays, however, he struck gold. He came across the online resource 'Help is at Hand', which has been developed by Keith Hawton from the University of Oxford.[4] This excellent online resource is supported by Public Health England and the UK National Suicide Prevention Alliance. It is comprehensive without being overwhelming, providing information about how someone may be feeling as well as offering practical support about how and who to tell about the death. It also gives specific advice for helping people who have had different connections with the person who has died.

It has an important section on the challenging issue of what to tell a child if their parent or someone close to them has died by suicide. A natural response is to protect the child from the truth of what happened. Of course, it depends on the age and degree of their understanding, and the decision clearly rests with the parent or carer, but it is usually better to tell the truth. It overcomes the risk of them finding out accidentally by some other means and it also gives them the chance to ask questions and for a trusted adult to reassure them. They could be experiencing such a wide range of feelings and emotions – from abandonment, to guilt, to shock or disbelief. You may also have to decide whether the child should view the body or attend the funeral. Again, these are difficult decisions that will depend on the child's age and understanding. It is always good to offer the child choice, if possible. Speaking personally, when Clare died, we decided not to bring my young daughter to the funeral. I regret this decision. Having discussed it with my daughter since, she wishes she had attended the funeral because, in her mind, it was a case of one day Clare was alive and then she didn't see her again. My daughter was confused by the experience, as well as being incredibly sad at losing Clare – she had no ending.

If you do decide that the child is too young to be told the truth, you can go back at a later date when they are older and gently explain what actually happened and why you told them a different story. There are also some really good books such as *Red Chocolate Elephants: For children bereaved by suicide* that can be helpful to support parents or other adults to have these sensitive conversations with children.[5] There are also specialist bereavement services and other organisations for children who are bereaved by suicide, which a GP should be able to signpost you to. If a sibling has died, in addition to the reactions already mentioned, the child may be left with unresolved issues, especially if they had a difficult relationship with their sibling who died. This may require careful support to help the young person work through these concerns.

It is also important to look out for friends and colleagues of the person who has died because they can feel overlooked or that they don't feel they have a right to grieve. Even though they may have shared a lifetime of experiences with them, they may feel excluded as they are not related. They may be devastated, also grieving, also struggling to make sense of what happened as they have also lost an important person in their life. It is essential that they are offered bereavement support if they need it. This point was also highlighted in the Suicide Bereavement UK survey. Those who had lost friends to suicide often reported feeling a disenfranchised or hidden grief, together with feelings of social isolation and being overlooked by services.

The impact of a death on friends is something I have really thought about since Clare died. I was fortunate, though. I was able to fly to Paris immediately after her death and support her husband Dave and spend the subsequent week with some of her family, trying to navigate Gallic bureaucracy to get her body repatriated. Although I hope I provided support to Dave, Clare's brother and her brother-in-law that week, it was so important for me and for my own grieving. I derived so much comfort from the time together with them in Paris. Over those five days, in between wails of tears and utter disbelief, we shared memories, celebrating Clare's life as well as mourning her passing. Although much of that week remains a blur, my memory is dominated by an early morning visit to the undertakers on the last day as Clare made her final journey home by plane.

I was extremely fortunate that I was able to help in the aftermath of Clare's death, but many other friends who are bereaved report different experiences. At a suicide bereavement conference, Linda, who lost her college friend Lee to suicide, told me that she is still angry with Lee's family. She felt that they had excluded her from the funeral arrangements. Part of her understands that this was simply because that is what happens when someone dies – it is for the family to organise the funeral. But she was angry because, according to her, they were best friends and, what is more, Lee had a really fractious relationship with his family. And it was her who had picked up all the pieces as he struggled through college. Even when I spoke to Linda two years on from the bereavement, she was still grieving Lee's loss and she remains adamant that what happened in the aftermath of Lee's death has hampered her ability to grieve. Irrespective of the specifics of Linda's experience, the wider point is that we should be mindful of people with different connections to the person who has died. They may need consideration and support irrespective of their relationship.

Returning to the 'Help is at Hand' guidance, I have summarised some of its key messages below to help support people, together with some of my reflections from speaking to people who have been bereaved. Each of the following is worth keeping in mind if someone you know has lost a loved one to suicide:

- We are all unique, therefore someone's experience of grief is unique.
- There is no set pathway through bereavement.
- Try not to tell someone how they should feel and, if you are bereaved, try to be patient if someone does, as they mean well.
- The pain of suicide loss can be felt acutely by those seemingly distant in relations from the person who has died (e.g., friends and colleagues).
- Feelings of grief can be overwhelming as well as being intertwined with moments of calmness.
- In the weeks and months following the death, it can be hard to predict the intensity of emotions. The only thing that is predictable is the unpredictability of grief.
- Feelings may range from anger to shock, guilt, shame, rejection, fear, loneliness, entrapment and stigma.
- Grief can affect someone physically, and may include palpitations, dizziness and headaches.
- Mental health can be affected, with people who are bereaved reporting depression, anxiety, post-traumatic stress and suicidal thoughts.
- In among the pain, some people report a sense of acceptance as their loved one is no longer suffering and it was their choice to end their life.

In terms of practical things that help, as Michael found, talking about thoughts and feelings is beneficial. But of course, everyone will find their own path in their own time. Initially Michael spoke to his close friends and family before reaching out to the SOBS group. Seeing a grief counsellor or a psychologist may suit others rather than attending a support group. Some people also find it helpful to make time to remember their loved one. This can take many different forms, but can include writing a journal, creating a memory box or visiting a special place. Others try to keep active and engage in self-care activities. Thinking about what isn't helpful, bottling up feelings, drinking more and not seeking help are probably top of the list of 'best to avoid'.

Being there for a relative or friend is key to helping someone who has been bereaved, making it clear to them that you are there for them whenever they would like to talk. Try to be non-judgemental, empathic and compassionate. As noted above, try not to tell them how they should be feeling because everyone's experience of grief is different. They should try to take each day as it comes. In terms of being there for them, they may simply need a sounding board for the questions that they have about the death or a space to share memories. Special dates like anniversaries and holidays can be particularly difficult. You may find it emotionally intense or draining, so it is important to look after yourself as well. If the person who is bereaved is a colleague returning to work after a death, it may be helpful to speak to them beforehand to see what they want you to do in terms of others knowing what happened. Again, the guiding principle is to respect their wishes; some may want other work colleagues to know and appreciate it when others acknowledge the death; conversely, they may want their privacy respected.

Although millions of people are newly bereaved by suicide each year, it is surprising that there is a real lack of research evidence for what is most effective to support people bereaved by suicide. In addition, the quality of many postvention studies remains low and the quantity of such studies is small. Postvention is the name for interventions to provide support to those bereaved by suicide. In 2019, Karl Andriessen and colleagues from the University of Melbourne published a review study of interventions for people bereaved by suicide, which also included grief, mental health or suicide-related outcomes.[6] Over a 35-year period, they could only find 11 studies that fitted their review criteria. Frustratingly, the findings were mixed. Whereas there was some support for general suicide grief interventions, the effectiveness of complicated grief interventions after suicide was weak. The interventions were often very different, which made it difficult to work out what may be effective. Some interventions were group-based, others were psychotherapeutic and the number of sessions also ranged from a single session to 16. On a more positive note however, these authors identified a few things that tended to be part of those interventions that were effective and they concluded that interventions that adopted a supportive, therapeutic and educational approach seemed to offer most promise. They also stressed the importance of interventions being led by trained facilitators, and they thought that the use of an intervention manual may be beneficial.

Although this review is welcome, it has given rise to more questions than answers about what works. For example, it is unclear whether interventions would be better delivered in a clinical setting versus someone's home or whether these interventions work for people across the lifespan, from different cultural backgrounds or from high-income versus low- or middle-income countries. Given that we know that people bereaved by suicide are at increased risk of suicide themselves, my plea is that research in this area gets the funding that it so badly needs.[7]

## Losing a Client or Patient to Suicide

If you are a mental health professional, you'll be aware of the impact of losing a patient or client to suicide. This is something that we have explored recently in a review of the research literature. Led by my colleague David Sandford, an experienced psychotherapist, we identified 54 studies that reported the impact of losing a patient to suicide on mental health professionals.[8] Similar to the effect on family and friends, across the studies the most common reactions felt by clinicians in interview-based studies were guilt, shock, sadness, anger and blame. Some of them also questioned why they hadn't seen the death coming. The impact was not only limited to personal reactions; the experience also contributed to self-doubt professionally. Some mental health professionals reported adopting a more cautious and defensive approach to the management of suicide risk. There was also evidence that as many as half of the clinicians in one study reported clinically significant levels of distress as a result of the trauma of losing a patient to suicide. A consistent conclusion across all of the studies was that more training on the impact of suicide was needed and that informal support was often cited as being beneficial.

As part of this programme of research, Dave also conducted in-depth interviews with mental health professionals to hear first-hand about the impact of the death of one of their patients.[9] Take Susan, a cognitive behavioural therapist with six years' experience – she highlights the traumatic nature and shock of discovering that someone she had recently worked with clinically had ended their life:

I was in shock and then I just started crying . . . Like with any traumatic event that you experience, it feels like it was only yesterday. I can remember exactly the day I found out . . . it did make me feel like I was responsible, even though I know I wasn't, you do feel like you're on trial.

Or Isabelle, who had been working as a psychological well-being practitioner for three years when she lost a client to suicide, who was also in shock:

It was a real shock, I found it really upsetting, more than I expected to be upset by . . . I remember feeling really kind of shaky, I felt physically sick.

The sense of responsibility she feels is also palpable:

. . . this was my case and he was my patient and I thought . . . I'm responsible for this young lad . . . I did feel a strong sense of responsibility for this young man. I just felt so sorry for his mother and obviously about him being so young. Oh my God, it's going to be awful, they're going to hold me responsible and rip me to pieces.

Although only female mental health practitioners took part in Dave's study, I know from speaking to male clinicians and the findings of our review study that male mental health practitioners report the same experiences. It is so important to remember that the causes of suicide are complex, therefore the responsibility for someone's death should never lie with one person. Though each of these reactions is understandable, they highlight the importance of self-care and the need for support for mental health practitioners who lose a patient to suicide. For precisely this purpose, a resource has been developed for psychiatrists, but which is applicable to all mental health professionals who lose a patient or client to suicide. The resource, developed by the Centre for Suicide Research at Oxford, highlights a range of strategies that may be helpful. It recommends that mental health professionals stay connected with the people around them in the short term after a death.[10] This should help to reduce the risk of them becoming isolated and give them the opportunities to avail of support from people they trust. Other strategies they describe include reminding practitioners to be self-compassionate, not to be too self-critical and not to blame themselves. It also emphasises the significance of focusing on their own emotional and physical health, together with the value in seeking both informal and formal help. It also suggests that mental health practitioners should consider temporarily adjusting their work patterns. The latter may help with recovery from the shock and trauma of the death, if necessary. The sad reality is that across their career, it is likely that most mental health professionals will lose a patient to suicide at some stage. And although each mental health practitioner's reaction will be different, if they do not look after their own well-being then they will be less able to help the very people who are most vulnerable.

Dealing with the aftermath of suicide is not limited to mental health care settings. The principles and concerns identified here are also applicable to professionals working across health, forensic, social care and educational settings. The devastation of a teacher, a social worker or a prison officer may be no less painful than a mental health clinician. We need to ensure that anyone who loses a client, a patient, a student or a prisoner to suicide is offered compassionate support as required.

# Epilogue

IN THIS BOOK I have tried to distil what I've learned both personally and professionally from my life so far in suicide prevention research. As I reflect on the past 12 months of writing, I am repeatedly drawn to the parallels with my own experience of personal therapy. In the early days of planning this book, I just couldn't settle upon what I wanted to say. I felt constrained and frustrated, struggling to find my own voice. Those feelings are reminiscent of the early days of my weekly 8am arrivals at my therapist's office. As I'd ascend the stairs of the imposing Victorian townhouse in Glasgow I'd get quite nervous. I'd repeatedly ask myself, 'What am I going to talk about for the next 50 minutes?' So I quickly learned to script myself, so that as soon as I entered the therapy room I was ready to go, feeling protected from enquiry and secure in keeping my distance from silence. Clearly this was a self-limiting strategy, but, at the time, it was my means of feeling secure and retaining my own sense of control over what I was willing to share.

It took me weeks to relinquish the protection of my mental script and to allow myself the space for things to bubble up. But when I did, I was able to better process what was contributing to my discontent, and to try to get to the heart of my own feelings of emptiness. This process feels very similar to how I have written this book. Initially, I was so frantic to commit words to the page that I didn't take the time to breathe, to allow the important things to bubble up to the surface. I'd focus in on some key facts around suicide prevention, as this was safe territory for me. But as days became weeks, and weeks became months, I became more confident. With this freedom, my own experiences were able to break through.

Nightly, I'd sit down in front of the computer, equipped only with a few sentences of overview, and I'd wait to see what emerged. Every so often a past encounter with someone who had been suicidal or bereaved would come to mind and it would help me to tell the story of how or why suicidal thoughts erupt in some but not in others. Or a memory would strike me as pertinent and allow me to convey what we need to do to prevent the needless loss of life or how to better support those left behind. I hope that by combining these personal recollections with the research evidence I've been able to provide a sense of the pain that those who are suicidal experience when they are at their darkest. Suicide is not a selfish act; for most, it is the ultimate act of despair.

I have also tried to dispel many of the myths that surround suicide, to illustrate the complex pathways from suicidal thoughts to suicidal acts and what works to prevent suicidal behaviour. In so doing, I have tried to provide hope. Hope for those who have been suicidal and hope for those who have been bereaved. Although we can never bring back those who we have lost, we can better support those left behind and, if we work together, we can save more lives. My ultimate hope is that, as a society, if we are kinder and more compassionate, both to ourselves and to those around us, then we will go some distance in protecting all of us from the devastation of suicide.

# Resources

BELOW ARE SOME helpful organisations for people in crisis or bereaved by suicide, both in the UK and internationally.

## UK Organisations

**NHS 111** is available to provide urgent care, advice and mental health support, day or night.
Phone: 111, every day, 24 hours a day
Website: www.111.nhs.uk

**Samaritans** is a voluntary organisation that offers support for anyone in distress.
Phone: 116 123, every day, 24 hours a day
Email: jo@samaritans.org
Website: www.samaritans.org

### Young people in crisis

**Childline** is a free helpline for anyone under 19 in the UK with any issue that they are going through.

Phone: 0800 1111, every day, 9am to 3:30am (the number doesn't show up on the phone bill)
Website: www.childline.org.uk

**The Mix** is an information and support service for young people (25 years and younger). It operates via an online community, on social, through a free, confidential helpline or a counselling service.
Phone: 0808 808 4994, every day, 3pm to midnight.
Crisis messenger text service: text 85258, every day, 24 hours a day
Website: www.themix.org.uk

**PAPYRUS** is a national charity dedicated to the prevention of young suicide. It operates **HOPELINEUK,** which offers support and advice to young people (under 35 years) at risk of suicide.
Phone: 0800 068 41 41, every day, 9am to midnight
Text: 0786 003 9967
Email: pat@papyrus-uk.org
Website: www.papyrus-uk.org

**Shout** is a free, confidential, 24/7 text messaging support service for anyone who is struggling to cope, anywhere, anytime.
Text: Shout to 85258
Website: www.giveusashout.org

**YoungMinds** aims to make sure all young people can get the mental health support they need, when they need it. The YoungMinds Crisis Messenger service is free 24/7 for young people experiencing a mental health crisis.
Text: YM to 85258

Phone: 0808 802 5544, Mon to Fri, 9.30am to 4pm, for parents needing help
Website: www.youngminds.org.uk

*Adults in crisis*

**4 Mental Health** is a group of professionals who have developed a range of mental health training programmes including safety planning resources.
Website: www.stayingsafe.net/home

**Age UK** provides services and support to older people.
Phone: 0800 678 1602, every day, 8am to 7pm
Website: www.ageuk.org.uk

**Breathing Space** (Scotland only) offers a free, confidential phone service for anyone in Scotland over the age of 16 experiencing low mood, depression or anxiety.
Phone: 0800 83 85 87, Mon to Thur, 6pm to 2am; Fri 6pm to Mon 6am
Website: www.breathingspace.scot

**CALM** exists to prevent male suicide in the UK. The helpline is free, anonymous and confidential.
Phone: 0800 58 58 58, every day, 5pm to midnight
Webchat: www.thecalmzone.net/help/webchat
Email: info@thecalmzone.net
Website: www.thecalmzone.net

**Lifeline** is the Northern Ireland crisis response helpline service for people who are experiencing distress or despair.

Phone: 0808 808 8000, every day, 24 hours a day
Website: www.lifelinehelpline.info

**Mind** provides advice and support to empower anyone experiencing a mental health problem.
Phone: 0300 123 3393, Mon to Fri, 9am to 6pm
Email: info@mind.org.uk
Website: www.mind.org.uk

**National Suicide Prevention Alliance (NSPA)** is an alliance of public, private and voluntary organisations in England to reduce suicide and support those bereaved or affected by suicide.
Website: https://www.nspa.org.uk

**SANEline** offers a national out-of-hours mental health helpline for anyone affected by mental illness, including family, friends and carers.
Phone: 0300 304 7000, every day, 4.30pm to 10.30pm
Email: support@sane.org.uk
Website: www.sane.org.uk

**Silver Line** is a free confidential helpline providing information, friendship and advice to older people.
Phone: 0800 4 70 80 90, every day, 24 hours a day
Website: www.thesilverline.org.uk

*Bereaved by suicide*

**Age UK** provides services and support to older people.
Phone: 0800 678 1602, every day, 8am to 7pm
Website: www.ageuk.org.uk

The **Bereavement Advice Centre** supports and advises people on what they need to do after a death.
Phone: 0800 634 9494, Mon to Fri, 9am to 5pm
Website: www.bereavementadvice.org

**Child Bereavement UK** aims to help children and young people (up to age 25), parents and families, to rebuild their lives when a child grieves or when a child dies.
Phone: 0800 02 888 40, Mon to Fri, 9am to 5pm
Email: support@childbereavementuk.org
Website: www.childbereavementuk.org

**Cruse Bereavement Care** offers support, advice and information to children, young people and adults when someone dies.
Phone: 0808 808 1677 – see website for operating times
Email: helpline@cruse.org.uk
Website: www.cruse.org.uk

**Support After Suicide Partnership** provides details of support for those bereaved or affected by suicide.
Website: www.supportaftersuicide.org.uk

**Survivors of Bereavement by Suicide (SOBS)** is a national charity providing dedicated support to adults who have been bereaved by suicide.
Phone: 0300 111 5065, every day, 9am to 9pm
Email: email.support@uksobs.org
Website: www.uk-sobs.org.uk

**The Compassionate Friends** provides support for those who lose a child from any cause.

Phone: 0345 123 2304, every day, 10am to 4pm and 7pm to 10pm
Email: helpline@tcf.org.uk
Website: www.tcf.org.uk

**Winston's Wish** provides support for bereaved children and families
Phone: 08088 020 021, Mon to Fri, 9am to 5pm
Email: chris@winstonswish.org.uk
Website: www.winstonswish.org.uk

## International Organisations

**Befrienders Worldwide** is an international network to provide emotional support services for people who are suicidal and/or in distress. The website includes useful information about international help and support.
Website: www.befrienders.org

The **International Association for Suicide Prevention (IASP)** hosts a database of organisations that provide crisis support in Africa, Asia, Europe, North America, Oceania and South America.
International Crisis Support: https://www.iasp.info/resources/Crisis_Centres

**Suicide.org** also maintains a database of international crisis helplines.
Website: www.suicide.org/international-suicide-hotlines.html

## Other Resources

**Building Suicide-Safer Schools and Colleges:** A guide for teachers and staff.
www.papyrus-uk.org/save-the-class

**#chatsafe:** Tools and tips to help young people communicate safely online about suicide and self-harm.
www.orygen.org.au/chatsafe

**Coping with Self-Harm:** A guide for parents and carers.
www.psych.ox.ac.uk/news/new-guide-for-parents-who-are-coping-with-their-child2019s-self-harm-2018you-are-not-alone2019

**Finding the Words:** How to support someone who has been bereaved and affected by suicide.
https://hub.supportaftersuicide.org.uk/resource/finding-the-words

**Help is at Hand:** Support after someone may have died by suicide. A resource for people who have been bereaved by suicide.
www.supportaftersuicide.org.uk/resource/help-is-at-hand

**If a Patient Dies by Suicide:** A resource for psychiatrists.
www.rcpsych.ac.uk/members/supporting-you/if-a-patient-dies-by-suicide

**National Collaborating Centre for Mental Health / NHS Health Education England:** Self-harm and suicide prevention

competency frameworks for supporting people who self-harm or are suicidal.
www.hee.nhs.uk/our-work/mental-health/self-harm-suicide-prevention-frameworks

**Suicide Bereavement UK:** Suicide bereavement training.
www.suicidebereavementuk.com

**Suicide Prevention Resource Center:** Hosts extensive information and resources for training in suicide prevention.
www.sprc.org

**The Art of Conversation:** A guide to talking, listening and reducing stigma surrounding suicide.
www.healthscotland.com/documents/2842.aspx

**Zero Suicide Alliance:** Online suicide awareness training.
www.zerosuicidealliance.com

# Acknowledgements

THIS BOOK WOULD not have been possible without the support, encouragement, insights and inspiration from so many family members, friends and colleagues.

I am particularly grateful to Andy Denholm, Ronan O'Carroll, Daryl O'Connor, Suzy O'Connor, Jane Pirkis, Alexandra Pitman, Steve Platt and Katie Robb, who read parts of the book at different stages of the writing process, and gave me invaluable and constructive feedback or fact-checked for me. Needless to say, any inaccuracies are all mine. To Seonaid Cleare and Karen Wetherall, who were welcome sounding boards at an early stage when I was trying to think through the book's structure. Thanks also to Will Storr, who generously provided me with advice about this author business.

I have also been incredibly lucky to have worked with so many fantastic people who have shaped my thinking, as well as many of them being long-standing collaborators. I'd like to acknowledge Chris Armitage, Clare Cassidy, Derek de Beurs, Eamon Ferguson, David Gunnell, Keith Hawton, Dave Jobes, Nav Kapur, Olivia Kirtley, Matt Nock, Ronan O'Carroll, Daryl O'Connor, Jane Pirkis, Steve Platt, Susan Rasmussen, Noel Sheehy, Ellen Townsend and Mark Williams. A huge thanks to all members, past and present, of the Suicidal Behaviour Research Lab. So much of the research that I have mentioned in this book was led by them; their energy, passion and enthusiasm continue to inspire me every day.

I am also indebted to all those who I've met along my journey, especially to those who have been bereaved or who have been suicidal. I have been humbled by your willingness to share something of your stories, of heartbreak as well as of hope, with me. I would also like to thank everyone who has taken part in our research studies over the past 25 years. It goes without saying that any progress that we have made is, in large part, thanks to your willingness to give so generously of your time.

This book may never have happened if it wasn't for a bit of serendipity. As I said in the Introduction, I had wanted to write this book for several years but I just couldn't settle on a structure or format. That was until July 2019 when I had a breakthrough, a eureka moment of sorts, one night while on holiday in Crete. I was able to visualise a way forward and resolved to contact potential publishers as soon as I got back to the UK. But here's the uncanny/spooky/serendipitous (delete as appropriate) coincidence without which this book may not have materialised. As I scrolled through the backlog of emails on the day of my return, nestled among them was an innocuous looking message entitled 'Book publishing – request' from Sara Cywinski, an editorial director from Penguin Random House. Initially, I scanned past it thinking it was probably a request for me to review a book proposal. Sara was on maternity leave at the time, but she had emailed as she was keen to get the ball rolling on some projects she'd like to explore on her return. And one of those was a book on suicide. I couldn't believe the coincidence or the timing. It was like a meeting of minds. I am so incredibly grateful to Sara, because in the subsequent weeks, she worked with me to structure the book and introduced me to Sam Jackson, Senior Commissioning Editor at Vermilion. Sam, together with Marta Catalano, has also been so supportive, expertly guiding me through to publication. I have also been so fortunate to have Julia Kellaway as my editor; her incisive but sensitive suggestions and edits have improved the book immeasurably.

Finally, this book would not have been possible without the unstinting support of Suzy, Poppy and Oisin, who have had to put up with me being holed up in the attic most evenings and weekends during the autumn and winter of 2020.

# Endnotes

## Part 1: Suicide: An Overview

1 World Health Organization (2018). World suicide prevention report.

2 Cerel, J., Brown, M. M., Maple, M., Singleton, M., Van de Venne, J., Moore, M., & Flaherty, C. (2019). How many people are exposed to suicide? Not six. *Suicide and Life-Threatening Behavior, 49,* 529–34.

3 McCrea, P. H. (1996). Trends in suicide in Northern Ireland 1922–1992. *Irish Journal of Psychological Medicine, 13,* 9–12; O'Neill, S., & O'Connor, R. C. (2020). Suicide in Northern Ireland: epidemiology, risk factors, and prevention. *Lancet Psychiatry, 7,* 538–546.

4 World Health Organization (2018). World suicide prevention report; World Health Organization (2019). Suicide in the world: Global health estimates.

## Chapter 1: The How, Who and When of Suicide

1 O'Connor, R. C., Sheehy, N. P., & O'Connor, D. B. (1999). A thematic suicide note analysis: Some observations on depression and previous suicide attempt. *Crisis, 20,* 106–14.

2 O'Connor, R. C., & Leenaars, A. A. (2004). A thematic comparison of suicide notes drawn from Northern Ireland and the United States. *Current Psychology*, *22*, 339–47.

3 O'Connor, R. C., & Nock, M. K. (2014). The psychology of suicidal behaviour. *Lancet Psychiatry*, *1*, 73–85.

4 Silverman, M. M. (2016). Challenges in defining and classifying suicide and suicidal behaviors. In: O'Connor, R. C., & Pirkis, J. (eds.) (2016). *The International Handbook of Suicide Prevention*. Wiley-Blackwell, 11–35; Siddaway, A. P., Wood, A. M., O'Carroll, R. E., & O'Connor, R. C. (2019). Characterizing self-injurious cognitions: Development and validation of the Suicide Attempt Beliefs Scale (SABS) and the Nonsuicidal Self-Injury Beliefs Scale (NSIBS). *Psychological Assessment, 31,* 592–608.

5 National Institute for Health and Care Excellence (2011). Self-harm in over 8s: Long-term management [clinical guideline CG133]. Retrieved from https://www.nice.org.uk/guidance/cg133 (accessed 10 Sept. 2020). (The self-harm management guidelines are currently being updated: National Institute for Health and Care Excellence (not yet published). Self-harm: Assessment, management and preventing recurrence [in development GID-NG10148]. Retrieved from https://www.nice.org.uk/guidance/indevelopment/gid-ng10148 (accessed 1 Feb. 2021).

6 Kapur, N., Cooper, J., O'Connor, R. C., & Hawton, K. (2013). Attempted suicide versus non-suicidal self injury: New diagnosis, or false dichotomy? *British Journal of Psychiatry*, *202*, 326–8.

7 World Health Organization (2018). Global health estimates 2016: Deaths by cause, age, sex, by country and by region, 2000–2016; World Health Organization (2 Sep. 2019). Suicide: Key facts. Retrieved from https://www.who.int/news-room/factsheets/detail/suicide (accessed 25 Nov. 2020).

8 Naghavi, M. (2019). Global, regional, and national burden of suicide mortality 1990 to 2016: Systematic analysis for the Global Burden of Disease Study 2016. *BMJ, 364*.

9 World Health Organization (2018). Global health estimates 2016: Deaths by cause, age, sex, by country and by region, 2000–2016; Vijaykumar, L., & Phillips, M. (2016). Suicide prevention in low- and middle-income countries. In: O'Connor, R. C., & Pirkis, J. (eds.) (2016). *The International Handbook of Suicide Prevention.* Wiley-Blackwell, 507–23; World Health Organization (2 Sep. 2019). Suicide: Key facts. Retrieved from https://www.who.int/news-room/fact-sheets/detail/suicide (accessed 25 Nov. 2020).

10 Turecki, G., Brent, D. A., Gunnell, D., O'Connor, R. C., Oquendo, M. A, Pirkis, J., & Stanley, B. H. (2019). Suicide and suicide risk. *Nature Reviews Disease Primers*, 5(74); Turecki, G., & Brent, D. A. (2016). Suicide and suicidal behaviour. *Lancet*, 387(10024), 1227–39; Hawton, K., Saunders, K. E. A., & O'Connor, R. C. (2012). Self-harm and suicide in adolescents. *Lancet*, 379, 2373–82.

11 National Center for Health Statistics (Apr. 2020). Increase in suicide mortality in the United States, 1999–2018. Retrieved from https://www.cdc.gov/nchs/products/databriefs/db362.htm (accessed 2 Jan. 2021); Office for National Statistics (3 Sep. 2019). Suicides in the UK: 2018 registrations. Retrieved from https://www.ons.gov.uk/peoplepopulationandcommunity/birthsdeathsandmarriages/deaths/bulletins/suicidesintheunitedkingdom/2018registrations (accessed 10 Oct. 2020).

12 Richardson, C., Robb, K. A., & O'Connor, R. C. (2020). A systematic review of suicidal behaviour in men: A narrative synthesis of risk factors. *Social Science & Medicine*; Scourfield, J., & Evans, R. (2015). Why might men be more at risk of suicide after a relationship breakdown? Sociological insights. *American Journal of Men's Health*, 9, 380–4; Scourfield, J., Fincham, B., Langer, S., & Shiner, M. (2012). Sociological autopsy: An integrated approach to the study of suicide in men. *Social Science & Medicine*, 74, 466–73; Canetto, S. S., & Cleary, A. (2012). Men, masculinities and suicidal behaviour. *Social Science & Medicine*, 74, 461–5;

Hunt, T., Wilson, C. J., Caputi, P., Woodward, A., & Wilson, I. (2017). Signs of current suicidality in men: A systematic review. *PLOS ONE*, *12*, e0174675.

13 The World Health Organization publishes the latest available international suicide rates: https://www.who.int/teams/mental-health-and-substance-use/suicide-data (accessed 27 Jan. 2021).

14 Naghavi, M. (2019). Global, regional, and national burden of suicide mortality 1990 to 2016: Systematic analysis for the Global Burden of Disease Study 2016. *BMJ*, *364*; World Health Organization (2018). Global health estimates 2016: Deaths by cause, age, sex, by country and by region, 2000–2016.

15 National Center for Health Statistics (Apr. 2020). Increase in suicide mortality in the United States, 1999–2018. Retrieved from https://www.cdc.gov/nchs/products/databriefs/db362.htm (accessed 2 Jan. 2021).

16 Office for National Statistics (3 Sep. 2019). Suicides in the UK: 2018 registrations. Retrieved from https://www.ons.gov.uk/peoplepopulationandcommunity/birthsdeathsandmarriages/deaths/bulletins/suicidesintheunitedkingdom/2018registrations (accessed 3 Nov. 2020); Samaritans (n.d.). Suicide facts and figures.Retrievedfromhttps://www.samaritans.org/scotland/about-samaritans/research-policy/suicide-facts-and-figures/ (accessed 26 May 2020).

17 Turecki, G., Brent, D. A., Gunnell, D., O'Connor, R. C., Oquendo, M. A, Pirkis, J., & Stanley, B. H. (2019). Suicide and suicide risk. *Nature Reviews Disease Primers*, *5*(74); Office for National Statistics (3 Sep. 2019). Suicides in the UK: 2018 registrations. Retrieved from https://www.ons.gov.uk/peoplepopulationandcommunity/birthsdeathsandmarriages/deaths/bulletins/suicidesintheunitedkingdom/2018registrations (accessed 3 Nov. 2020).

18 Naghavi, M. (2019). Global, regional, and national burden of suicide mortality 1990 to 2016: Systematic analysis for the Global Burden of Disease Study 2016. *BMJ*, *364*.

19 World Health Organization (2014). Preventing suicide: A global imperative.

20 Arensman, E., Griffin, E., & Corcoran, P. (2016). Self-harm: Extent of the problem and prediction of repetition. In: O'Connor, R. C., & Pirkis, J. (eds.) (2016). *The International Handbook of Suicide Prevention*. Wiley-Blackwell, 61–73.

21 Hawton, K., Saunders, K. E. A, & O'Connor, R. C. (2012). Self-harm and suicide in adolescents. *Lancet, 379*, 2373–82; Gillies, D., Christou, M. A., Dixon, A. C., Featherston, O. J., Rapti, I., Garcia-Anguita, A., Villasis-Keever, M., Reebye, P., Christou, E., & Al Kabir, N. (2018). Prevalence and characteristics of self-harm in adolescents: Meta-analyses of community-based studies 1990–2015. *Journal of the American Academy of Child & Adolescent Psychiatry, 57*, 733–41.

22 Uddin, R., Burton, N. W., Maple, M., Khan, S. R., & Khan, A. (2019). Suicidal ideation, suicide planning, and suicide attempts among adolescents in 59 low-income and middle-income countries: A population-based study. *Lancet Child & Adolescent Health, 3*, 223–33.

23 Cabello, M., Miret, M., Ayuso-Mateos, J. L., Caballero, F. F., Chatterji, S., Tobiasz-Adamczyk, B., Haro, J. M., Koskinen, S., Leonardi, M., & Borges, G. (2020). Cross-national prevalence and factors associated with suicide ideation and attempts in older and young-and-middle age people. *Aging & Mental Health, 24*, 1533–42.

24 Nock, M. K., Borges, G., Bromet, E. J., . . . & Williams, D. (2008). Cross-national prevalence and risk factors for suicidal ideation, plans and attempts. *British Journal of Psychiatry, 192*, 98–105.

25 di Giacomo, E., Krausz, M., Colmegna, F., Aspesi, F., & Clerici, M. (2019). Estimating the risk of attempted suicide among sexual minority youths: A systematic review and meta-analysis. *JAMA Pediatrics, 172*, 1145–52; Glenn, C. R., Kleiman, E. M., Kellerman,

J., Pollak, O., Cha, C. B., Esposito, E. C., Porter, A. C., Wyman, P. A., & Boatman, A. E. (2020). Annual research review: A meta-analytic review of worldwide suicide rates in adolescents. *Journal of Child Psychology and Psychiatry*, *61*, 294–308; McNeil, J., Ellis, S. J., & Eccles, F. J. R. (2017). Suicide in trans populations: A systematic review of prevalence and correlates. *Psychology of Sexual Orientation and Gender Diversity*, *4*, 341–53.

26 Platt, S. (2016). Inequalities and suicidal behavior. In: O'Connor, R. C., & Pirkis, J. (eds.) (2016). *The International Handbook of Suicide Prevention*. Wiley-Blackwell, 258–83.

27 Holmes, E. A., O'Connor, R. C., Perry, V. H., Wesseley, S., Arseneault, L., Ballard, C., Christensen, H., Cohen Silver, R., Everall, I., Ford, T., John, A., Kabir, T., King, K., Madan, I., Michie, S., Przybylski, A. K., Shafran, R., Sweeney, A., Worthman, C. M., Yardley, L., Cowan, K., Cope, C., Hotopf, M., & Bullmore, E. (2020). Multidisciplinary research priorities for the COVID-19 pandemic: A call for action for mental health science. *Lancet Psychiatry*, *7*, 547–60.

28 Gunnell, D., Appleby, L., Arensman, E., Hawton, K., John, A., Kapur, N., Khan, M., O'Connor, R. C., Pirkis, J., & the COVID-19 Suicide Prevention Research Collaboration. (2020). Suicide risk and prevention during the COVID-19 pandemic. *Lancet Psychiatry*, *7*, 468–71; Moutier, C. (2020). Suicide prevention in the COVID-19 era: Transforming threat into opportunity. *JAMA Psychiatry*.

29 Yip, P. S., Cheung, Y. T., Chau, P. H., & Law, Y. W. (2010). The impact of epidemic outbreak: The case of severe acute respiratory syndrome (SARS) and suicide among older adults in Hong Kong. *Crisis*, *31*, 86–92.

30 Reeves, A., McKee, M., & Stuckler, D. (2014). Economic suicides in the Great Recession in Europe and North America. *British Journal of Psychiatry*, *205*, 246–7.

31 Czeisler, M. É., Lane, R. I., Petrosky, E., Wiley, J. F., Christensen, A., Njai, R., Weaver, M. D., Robbins, R., Facer-Childs, E. R.,

Barger, L. K., Czeisler, C. A., Howard, M. E., & Rajaratnam, S. (2020). Mental health, substance use, and suicidal ideation during the COVID-19 Pandemic – United States, June 24–30, 2020. *MMWR. Morbidity and Mortality Weekly Report*, 69, 1049–57.

32 O'Connor, R. C., Wetherall, K., Cleare, S., McClelland, H., Melson, A. J., Niedzwiedz, C. L., O'Carroll, R. E., O'Connor, D. B., Platt, S., Scowcroft, E., Watson, B., Zortea, T., Ferguson, E., & Robb, K. A. (2020). Mental health and wellbeing during the COVID-19 pandemic: Longitudinal analyses of adults in the UK COVID-19 Mental Health & Wellbeing study. *British Journal of Psychiatry*.

33 Niederkrotenthaler, T., Gunnell, D., Arensman, E., Pirkis, J., Appleby, L., Hawton, K., John, A., Kapur, N., Khan, M., O'Connor, R. C., Platt, S., & the International COVID-19 Suicide Prevention Research Collaboration (2021). Suicide research, prevention, and COVID-19. Towards a global response and the establishment of an international research collaboration. *Crisis, 41*, 321–30; John, A., Pirkis, J., Gunnell, D., Appleby, L., & Morrissey, J. (2020). Trends in suicide during the COVID-19 pandemic. *BMJ*, *371*,m4352; Tanaka, T., & Okamoto, S. (2021). Increase in suicide following an initial decline during the COVID-19 pandemic in Japan. *Nature Human Behavior*.

34 Galasinski, D. (21 Jun. 2019). Re-visiting language and suicide [blog]. Retrieved from https://dariuszgalasinski.com/2019/06/21/language-and-suicide-2/#more-2280 (accessed 25 Sep. 2020).

35 Rasmussen, S., Hawton, K., Philpott-Morgan, S., & O'Connor, R. C. (2016). Why do adolescents self-harm? An investigation of motives in a community sample. *Crisis, 37*, 176–83; de Beurs, D., Vancayseele, N., van Borkulo, C., Portzky, G., & van Heeringen, K. (2018). The association between motives, perceived problems and current thoughts of self-harm following an episode of self-harm. A network analysis. *Journal of Affective Disorders*, 240, 262–70.

36  Padmanathan, P., Biddle, L., Hall, K., Scowcroft, E., Nielsen, E.,
&  Knipe, D. (2019). Language use and suicide: An online cross-
sectional survey. *PLOS ONE*, *14*, e0217473.

# Chapter 2: What Suicidal Pain Feels Like

1  Leenaars, A. A., Dieserud, G., Wenckstern, S., Dyregrov, K., Lester,
D., & Lyke, J. (2018). A multidimensional theory of suicide. *Crisis*, *39*, 416–27.

2  Turecki, G., Brent, D. A., Gunnell, D., O'Connor, R. C., Oquendo,
M. A, Pirkis, J., & Stanley, B. H. (2019). Suicide and suicide
risk. *Nature Reviews Disease Primers*, *5*(74).

3  O'Connor, R. C., Sheehy, N. P., & O'Connor, D. B. (1999). A
thematic suicide note analysis: Some observations on depression
and previous suicide attempt. *Crisis*, *20*, 106–14.

4  National Confidential Inquiry into Suicide and Safety in Mental
Health (Dec. 2019). Annual report 2019: England, Northern Ireland, Scotland and Wales. Retrieved from https://sites.manchester.
ac.uk/ncish/reports/annual-report-2019-england-northern-
ireland-scotland-and-wales/ (accessed 9 July. 2020).

5  Walker, M. (2018). *Why We Sleep*. Penguin.

6  Hysing, M., Sivertsen, B., Morten Stormark, K., & O'Connor,
R. C. (2015). Sleep problems and self-harm in adolescence. *British Journal of Psychiatry*, *207*, 306–12.

7  Liu, R. T., Steele, S. J., Hamilton, J. L., Quyen, B. P., Furbish, K.,
Burke, T. A., Martinez, A. P., & Gerlush, N. (2020). Sleep and sui-
cide: A systematic review and meta-analysis of longitudinal studies.
*Clinical Psychology Review*, *81*, 101895; Russell, K., Allan, S.,
Beattie, L., Bohan, J., MacMahon, K., & Rasmussen, S. (2019).
Sleep problem, suicide and self-harm in university students: A sys-
tematic review. *Sleep Medicine Reviews*, *44*, 58–69; Pigeon, W. R.,

Bishop, T. M., & Titus, C.E. (2016). The relationship between sleep disturbance, suicidal ideation, suicide attempts, and suicide among adults: A systematic review. *Psychiatric Annals, 46*, 177–86.

8  Shneidman, E. (1996). *The Suicidal Mind*. Oxford University Press.

9  Williams, M. (1997). *Cry of Pain: Understanding Suicide and Self-Harm*. Penguin; O'Connor, R. C., & Portzky, G. (2018). The relationship between entrapment and suicidal behavior through the lens of the integrated motivational–volitional model of suicidal behavior. *Current Opinion in Psychology, 22*, 12–17; Taylor, P. J., Gooding, P., Wood, A. M., & Tarrier, N. (2011). The role of defeat and entrapment in depression, anxiety, and suicide. *Psychological Bulletin, 137*, 391–420.

10  Kavalidou, K., Smith, D., & O'Connor, R. C. (2017). The role of physical and mental health multimorbidity in suicidal ideation. *Journal of Affective Disorders, 209*, 82–5.

11  Naroll, R. (1969). Cultural determinants and the concept of the sick society. In: Plog, S. C., & Edgerton, R. B. (eds.) (1969). *Changing Perspectives in Mental Illness*. Rinehart and Winston, 128–55.

12  International Association for Suicide Prevention (n.d.). World Suicide Prevention Day: Impact report. Retrieved from https://www.iasp.info/pdf/WSPD_2020_impact_report.pdf  (accessed 14 Dec. 2020).

## Chapter 3: Myths and Misunderstandings

1  Turecki, G., & Brent, D. A. (2016). Suicide and suicidal behaviour. *Lancet, 387*(10024), 1227–39; O'Connor, R. C., & Nock, M. K. (2014). The psychology of suicidal behaviour. *Lancet Psychiatry, 1*, 73–85.

2  O'Connor, R. C., & Sheehy, N. P (1997). Suicide and gender. *Mortality, 2*, 239–54.

3 Cavanagh, J., Carson, A., Sharpe, M., & Lawrie, S. (2003). Psychological autopsy studies of suicide: A systematic review. *Psychological Medicine, 33*, 395–405; Vijayakumar, L. (2005). Suicide and mental disorders in Asia. *International Review of Psychiatry, 17*, 109–14; Phillips, M. R., Yang, G., Zhang, Y., Wang, L., Ji, H., & Zhou, M. (2002). Risk factors for suicide in China: A national case-control psychological autopsy study. *Lancet, 360* (9347), 1728–36.

4 Hjelmeland, H., & Knizek, B. L. (2017). Suicide and mental disorders: A discourse of politics, power, and vested interests. *Death Studies, 41*, 481–92.

5 Turecki, G., Brent, D. A., Gunnell, D., O'Connor, R. C., Oquendo, M. A, Pirkis, J., & Stanley, B. H. (2019). Suicide and suicide risk. *Nature Reviews Disease Primers, 5*(74); Too, L. S., Spittal, M. J., Bugeja, L., Reifels, L., Butterworth, P., & Pirkis, J. (2019). The association between mental disorders and suicide: A systematic review and meta-analysis of record linkage studies. *Journal of Affective Disorders, 259*, 302–313.

6 O'Connor, R. C., & Nock, M. K. (2014). The psychology of suicidal behaviour. *Lancet Psychiatry, 1*, 73–85; van Heeringen, K. (2001). Towards a psychobiological model of the suicidal process. In: van Heeringen, K. (ed.) (2001). *Understanding Suicidal Behaviour*. John Wiley & Sons.

7 Vijaykumar, L., & Phillips, M. (2016). Suicide prevention in low- and middle-income countries. In: O'Connor, R. C., & Pirkis, J. (eds.) (2016). *The International Handbook of Suicide Prevention*. Wiley-Blackwell, 507–23.

8 Naghavi, M. (2019). Global, regional, and national burden of suicide mortality 1990 to 2016: Systematic analysis for the Global Burden of Disease Study 2016. *BMJ, 364*; World Health Organization (2018). Global Health Estimates 2016: Deaths by cause, age, sex, by country and by region, 2000–2016.

9 Shneidman, E. (1996). *The Suicidal Mind*. Oxford University Press.

10 Franklin, J. C., Ribeiro, J. D., Fox, K. R., Bentley, K. H., Kleiman, E. M., Huang, X., Musacchio, K. M., Jaroszewski, A. C., Chang, B. P., & Nock, M. K. (2017). Risk factors for suicidal thoughts and behaviors: A meta-analysis of 50 years of research. *Psychological Bulletin, 143,* 187–232.

11 Dazzi, T., Gribble, R., Wessely, S., & Fear, N. T. (2014). Does asking about suicide and related behaviours induce suicidal ideation? What is the evidence? *Psychological Medicine, 44,* 3361–3.

12 Shneidman, E. S. (1985). *Definition of Suicide.* John Wiley & Sons.

13 Kevin Hines's website describes his journey to recovery as well as other useful suicide prevention resources: http://www.kevinhinesstory.com (accessed 15 Aug. 2020).

14 Tidemalm, D., Runeson, B., Waern, M., Frisell, T., Carlström, E., Lichtenstein, P., & Långström, N. (2011). Familial clustering of suicide risk: A total population study of 11.4 million individuals. *Psychological Medicine, 41,* 2527–34; Fu, Q., Heath, A. C., Bucholz, K. K., Nelson, E. C., Glowinski, A. L., Goldberg, J., Lyons, M. J., Tsuang, M. T., Jacob, T., True, M. R., & Eisen, S. A. (2002). A twin study of genetic and environmental influences on suicidality in men. *Psychological Medicine, 32,* 11–24.

15 O'Connor, R. C., Rasmussen, S., Miles, J., & Hawton, K. (2009). Deliberate self-harm in adolescents: Self-report survey in schools in Scotland. *British Journal of Psychiatry, 194,* 68–72; O'Connor, R. C., Rasmussen, S., & Hawton, K. (2014). Adolescent self-harm: A school-based study in Northern Ireland. *Journal of Affective Disorders, 159,* 46–52.

16 Hawton, K., Saunders, K. E., & O'Connor, R. C. (2012). Self-harm and suicide in adolescents. *Lancet, 379,* 2373–82; Madge, N., Hawton, K., McMahon, E. M., Corcoran, P., De Leo, D., de Wilde, E. J., Fekete, S., van Heeringen, K., Ystgaard, M., & Arensman, E. (2011). Psychological characteristics, stressful life events and deliberate self-harm: Findings from the Child &

Adolescent Self-harm in Europe (CASE) Study. *European Child & Adolescent Psychiatry*, *20*, 499–508.

17 O'Connor, R. C., & Nock, M. K. (2014). The psychology of suicidal behaviour. *Lancet Psychiatry*, *1*, 73–85; Turecki, G., Brent, D. A., Gunnell, D., O'Connor, R. C., Oquendo, M. A, Pirkis, J., & Stanley, B. H. (2019). Suicide and suicide risk. *Nature Reviews Disease Primers*, *5*(74); Stack S. (2000). Suicide: A 15-year review of the sociological literature. Part I: Cultural and economic factors. *Suicide & Life-Threatening Behavior*, *30*, 145–62; Scourfield, J., Fincham, B., Langer, S., & Shiner, M. (2012). Sociological autopsy: An integrated approach to the study of suicide in men. *Social Science & Medicine*, *74*, 466–73; Colucci, E. (2013). Culture, cultural meaning(s), and suicide. In: Colucci, E., & Lester, D. (eds.), & Hjelmeland, H., & Park, B. C. B. (cols.) (2012). *Suicide and Culture: Understanding the Context*. Hogrefe Publishing, 25–46.

18 Zalsman, G., Hawton, K., Wasserman, D., van Heeringen, K., Arensman, E., Sarchiapone, M., Carli, V., Höschl, C., Barzilay, R., Balazs, J., Purebl, G., Kahn, J. P., Sáiz, P. A., Lipsicas, C. B., Bobes, J., Cozman, D., Hegerl, U., & Zohar, J. (2016). Suicide prevention strategies revisited: 10-year systematic review. *Lancet Psychiatry*, *3*, 646–59; the World Health Organization has also published a really helpful document on 'national suicide prevention strategies', which includes details of progress, examples and indicators: https://apps.who.int/iris/bitstream/handle/10665/279765/9789241515016-eng.pdf (accessed 10 Jan. 2021).

19 Naghavi, M. (2019). Global, regional, and national burden of suicide mortality 1990 to 2016: Systematic analysis for the Global Burden of Disease Study 2016. *BMJ*, *364*.

20 Scotland's recent suicide rates and suicide prevention action plans are available online: https://www.gov.scot/policies/mental-health/suicide (accessed 12 Jan. 2021).

21 Franklin, J. C., Ribeiro, J. D., Fox, K. R., Bentley, K. H., Kleiman, E. M., Huang, X., Musacchio, K. M., Jaroszewski, A. C.,

Chang, B. P., & Nock, M. K. (2017). Risk factors for suicidal thoughts and behaviors: A meta-analysis of 50 years of research. *Psychological Bulletin*, *143*, 187–232.

22  Platt, S. (2016). Inequalities and suicidal behavior. In: O'Connor, R. C., & Pirkis, J. (eds.) (2016). *The International Handbook of Suicide Prevention*. Wiley-Blackwell, 258–83.

23  Nock, M. K., Borges, G., Bromet, E. J., . . . & Williams, D. (2008). Cross-national prevalence and risk factors for suicidal ideation, plans and attempts. *British Journal of Psychiatry*, *192*, 98–105.

24  O'Connor, R. C., Wetherall, K., Cleare, S., Eschle, S., Drummond, J., Ferguson, E., O'Connor, D. B., & O'Carroll, R. E. (2018). Suicide attempts and non-suicidal self-harm: A national prevalence study of young adults. *British Journal of Psychiatry Open*, *4*, 142–8.

25  Hawton, K., Bergen, H., Kapur, N., Cooper, J., Steeg, S., Ness, J., & Waters, K. (2012). Repetition of self-harm and suicide following self-harm in children and adolescents: Findings from the Multicentre Study of Self-harm in England. *Journal of Child Psychology and Psychiatry and Allied Disciplines*, *53*, 1212–19.

# Chapter 4: Making Sense of a Suicide

1  Borges, G., Bagge, C. L., Cherpitel, C. J., Conner, K. R., Orozco, R., & Rossow, I. (2017). A meta-analysis of acute use of alcohol and the risk of suicide attempt. *Psychological Medicine*, *47*, 949–57.

2  Shneidman, E. (1996). *The Suicidal Mind*. Oxford University Press.

3  McDermott, L. (2016). An interpretative phenomenological analysis of the lived experience of suicidal behaviour [D Clin Psy thesis]. University of Glasgow. Retrieved from http://theses.gla.ac.uk/7569 (accessed 20 Oct. 2020).

4 Hawton, K., Saunders, K. E. A., & O'Connor, R. C. (2012). Self-harm and suicide in adolescents. *Lancet*, *379*, 2373–82.

5 Joiner, T. (2007). *Why People Die By Suicide*. Harvard University Press.

6 O'Connor, R. C., & Nock, M. K. (2014). The psychology of suicidal behaviour. *Lancet Psychiatry*, *1*, 73–85.

## Chapter 5: What Suicide is Not

1 O'Connor, R. C., & Nock, M. K. (2014). The psychology of suicidal behaviour. *Lancet Psychiatry*, *1*, 73–85.

2 World Health Organization/International Association for Suicide Prevention (2017). Media guidelines. Retrieved from https://www.iasp.info/media_guidelines.php (accessed 9 Jan. 2021).

3 Turecki, G., Brent, D. A., Gunnell, D., O'Connor, R. C., Oquendo, M. A, Pirkis, J., & Stanley, B. H. (2019). Suicide and suicide risk. *Nature Reviews Disease Primers*, *5*(74).

4 O'Connor, R. C. (1999). The boundaries: Health psychology and suicidal behaviour. *Health Psychology Update*, *36*, 4–7.

5 Bostwick, J. M., & Pankratz, V. S. (2000). Affective disorders and suicide risk: A reexamination. *American Journal of Psychiatry*, *157*, 1925–32.

6 Quinn, F., Chater, A., & Morrison, V. (2020). An oral history of health psychology in the UK. *British Journal of Health Psychology*, *25*, 502–18.

7 Conner, M., & Norman, P. (2005). *Predicting Health Behaviour*. Open University Press.

8 The International Association for Suicide Prevention has a task force on the decriminalisation of suicide: https://www.iasp.info/decriminalisation.php (accessed 18 Jan. 2021); Mishara, B. L.,

Weisstub, D.N. (2016). The legal status of suicide: a global review. International Journal of Law and Psychiatry 44, 54–74.

9 O'Connor, R. C. & Sheehy, N. P (1997). Suicide and gender. *Mortality*, 2, 239–54.

## Chapter 6: Towards An Integrated Understanding of Suicide

1 O'Connor, R. C., Platt, S., & Gordon, J. (eds.) (2011). *The International Handbook of Suicide Prevention: Research, Evidence and Practice.* Wiley-Blackwell.

2 Platt, S. (1984). Unemployment and suicidal behaviour: A review of the literature. *Social Science & Medicine, 19,* 93–115.

3 O'Connor, R. C. (2011). Towards an integrated motivational–volitional of suicidal behaviour. In: O'Connor, R. C., Platt, S., & Gordon, J. (eds.) (2011). *The International Handbook of Suicide Prevention: Research, Policy and Practice.* Wiley Blackwell, 181–98; O'Connor, R. C. (2011). The integrated motivational–volitional model of suicidal behaviour. *Crisis, 32,* 295–8.

4 Shneidman, E., & Farberow, N. (1957) *Clues to Suicide.* McGraw-Hill Book Company; Shneidman, E. (1967). *Essays in Self-destruction.* Science House; Baumeister, R. F. (1990). Suicide as escape from self. *Psychological Review, 97,* 90–113.

5 Baechler, J. (1979). *Suicides.* Basic Books; Baechler, J. (1980). A strategic theory. *Suicide and Life-Threatening Behavior, 10,* 70–99; Shneidman, E. (1996). *The Suicidal Mind.* Oxford University Press.

6 Williams, M. (1997). *Cry of Pain: Understanding Suicide and Self-Harm.* Penguin; Williams, J. M. G., Crane, C., Barnhofer, T., & Duggan, D. S. (2005). Psychology and suicidal behaviour: Elaborating the entrapment model. In: Hawton, K. (ed.) (2005).

*Prevention and Treatment of Suicidal Behaviour.* Oxford University Press, 71–90.

7 Gilbert, P., & Allan, S. (1998). The role of defeat and entrapment (arrested flight) in depression: An exploration of an evolutionary view. *Psychological Medicine, 28,* 585–98.

8 MacLean, P. D. (1990). *The Triune Brain in Evolution.* Plenum Press.

9 Gilbert, P., & Allan, S. (1998). The role of defeat and entrapment (arrested flight) in depression: An exploration of an evolutionary view. *Psychological Medicine, 28,* 585–98.

10 O'Connor, R. C., Smyth, R., Ferguson, E., Ryan, C., & Williams, J. M. G. (2013). Psychological processes and repeat suicidal behavior: A four year prospective study. *Journal of Consulting & Clinical Psychology, 81,* 1137–43.

11 O'Connor, R. C., & Portzky, G. (2018). The relationship between entrapment and suicidal behavior through the lens of the integrated motivational–volitional model of suicidal behavior. *Current Opinion in Psychology, 22,* 12–17; Taylor, P. J., Gooding, P., Wood, A. M., & Tarrier, N. (2011). The role of defeat and entrapment in depression, anxiety, and suicide. *Psychological Bulletin, 137,* 391–420; Siddaway, A. P., Taylor, P. J., Wood, A. M., & Schulz, J. (2015). A meta-analysis of perceptions of defeat and entrapment in depression, anxiety problems, posttraumatic stress disorder, and suicidality. *Journal of Affective Disorders, 184,* 149–59.

12 De Beurs, D., Cleare, S., Wetherall, K., Eschle-Byrne, S., Ferguson, E., O'Connor, D. B., & O'Connor, R. C. (2020). Entrapment and suicide risk: The development of the 4-item Entrapment Scale Short-Form (E-SF). *Psychiatry Research, 284,* 112765.

13 Wetherall, K., Cleare, S., Eschle, S., Ferguson, E., O'Connor, D. B., O'Carroll, R. E., & O'Connor, R. C. (2020). Predicting suicidal ideation in a nationally representative sample of young adults: A 12 month prospective study. *Psychological Medicine.*

14 Morrison, R., & O'Connor, R. C. (2008). A systematic review of the relationship between rumination and suicidality. *Suicide and Life-Threatening Behavior*, *38*, 523–38; Law, K. C., & Tucker, R. P. (2018). Repetitive negative thinking and suicide: A burgeoning literature with need for further exploration. *Current Opinion in Psychology*, *22*, 68–72.

15 Camus, A. (1985). *The Myth of Sisyphus*. Penguin.

16 Haig, M. (2015). *Reasons to Stay Alive*. Canongate.

17 Steele, C. M., & Josephs, R. A. (1990). Alcohol myopia: Its prized and dangerous effects. *American Psychologist*, *45*, 921–33.

18 Richardson, C., Robb, K. A., & O'Connor, R. C. (2020). A systematic review of suicidal behaviour in men: A narrative synthesis of risk factors. *Social Science & Medicine*.

19 Honeyman, G. (2018). *Eleanor Oliphant is Completely Fine*. HarperCollins.

# Chapter 7: The Integrated Motivational– Volitional Model of Suicidal Behaviour

1 O'Connor, R. C. (2011). Towards an integrated motivational– volitional of suicidal behaviour. In: O'Connor, R. C., Platt, S., & Gordon, J. (eds.) (2011). *The International Handbook of Suicide Prevention: Research, Policy and Practice*. Wiley Blackwell, 181–98; de Beurs, D. P., van Borkulo, C. D., & O'Connor, R. C. (2017). Association between suicidal symptoms and repeat suicidal behaviour within a sample of hospital-treated suicide attempters. *BJPsych Open*, *3*, 120–6.

2 O'Connor, R. C., & Kirtley, O. J. (2018). The integrated motivational–volitional model of suicidal behaviour. *Philosophical Transactions of the Royal Society B.*, *373*, 20170268.

3 O'Connor, R. C. (2011). Towards an integrated motivational–volitional of suicidal behaviour. In: O'Connor, R. C., Platt, S., & Gordon, J. (eds.) (2011). *The International Handbook of Suicide Prevention: Research, Policy and Practice*. Wiley Blackwell, 181–98.

4 Williams, M. (1997). *Cry of Pain: Understanding Suicide and Self-Harm*. Penguin; Gilbert, P., & Allan, S. (1998). The role of defeat and entrapment (arrested flight) in depression: An exploration of an evolutionary view. *Psychological Medicine, 28*, 585–98.

5 Joiner, T. (2007). *Why People Die By Suicide*. Harvard University Press; van Orden, K. A., Witte, T. K., Cukrowicz, K. C., Braithwaite, S. R., Selby, E. A., & Joiner, T. E., Jr (2010). The interpersonal theory of suicide. *Psychological Review, 117*, 575–600; Chu, C., Buchman-Schmitt, J. M., Stanley, I. H., Hom, M. A., Tucker, R. P., Hagan, C. R., Rogers, M. L., Podlogar, M. C., Chiurliza, B., Ringer, F. B., Michaels, M. S., Patros, C., & Joiner, T. E. (2017). The interpersonal theory of suicide: A systematic review and meta-analysis of a decade of cross-national research. *Psychological Bulletin, 143*, 1313–45.

6 Armitage, C. J., & Conner, M. (2001). Efficacy of the theory of planned behaviour: A meta-analytic review. *British Journal of Social Psychology, 40*, 471–99.

7 O'Connor, R. C., Armitage, C. J., & Gray, L. (2006). The role of clinical and social cognitive variables in parasuicide. *British Journal of Clinical Psychology, 45*, 465–81.

8 Ibid.

9 O'Connor, R. C. (2007). The relations between perfectionism and suicide risk: A systematic review. *Suicide and Life-Threatening Behavior, 37*, 698–714; Smith, M. M., Sherry, S. B., Checn, S., Saklofske, D. H., Mushquash, C., Flett, G. L., & Hewitt, P. L. (2018). The perniciousness of perfectionism: A meta-analytic review of the perfectionism–suicide relationship. *Journal of Personality, 86*, 522–42.

10  Turecki, G., Brent, D. A., Gunnell, D., O'Connor, R. C., Oquendo, M. A, Pirkis, J., & Stanley, B. H. (2019). Suicide and suicide risk. *Nature Reviews Disease Primers*, 5(74).

11  Ibid.

12  Stone, M., Laughren, T., Jones, M. L., Levenson, M., Holland, P. C., Hughes, A., Hammad, T. A., Temple, R., & Rochester, G. (2009). Risk of suicidality in clinical trials of antidepressants in adults: Analysis of proprietary data submitted to US Food and Drug Administration. *BMJ*, 339, b2880.

13  O'Connor, R. C., Whyte, M. C., Fraser, L., Masterton, G., & MacHale, S. (2007). Predicting short-term improvement in well-being following presentation to hospital with self-harm: The conjoint effects of social perfectionism and future thinking. *Behaviour Research and Therapy*, 45, 1543–55; O'Connor, R. C. (2007). The relations between perfectionism and suicide risk: A systematic review. *Suicide and Life-Threatening Behavior*, 37, 698–714; O'Connor, R. C., Rasmussen, S., & Hawton, K. (2010). Predicting depression, anxiety and self-harm in adolescents: The role of perfectionism and stress. *Behaviour Research and Therapy*, 48, 52–9.

14  O'Connor, R. C. (2007). The relations between perfectionism and suicide risk: A systematic review. *Suicide and Life-Threatening Behavior*, 37, 698–714; Smith, M. M., Sherry, S. B., Checn, S., Saklofske, D. H., Mushquash, C., Flett, G. L., & Hewitt, P. L. (2018). The perniciousness of perfectionism: A meta-analytic review of the perfectionism–suicide relationship. *Journal of Personality*, 86, 522–42; Roxborough, H. M., Hewitt, P. L., Kaldas, J., Flett, G. L., Caelian, C. M., Sherry, S., & Sherry, D. L. (2012). Perfectionistic self-presentation, socially prescribed perfectionism, and suicide in youth: A test of the perfectionism social disconnection model. *Suicide & Life-threatening Behavior*, 42, 217–33.

15  Storr, W. (2017). *Selfie: How the West Became Self-Obsessed*. Picador; Storr, W. (11 May 2015). The male suicides: How social

perfectionism kills. Mosaic Science. Retrieved from https://mosaicscience.com/story/male-suicide (accessed 9 Jan. 2021).

16 Hewitt, P. L., & Flett, G. L. (1991). Perfectionism in the self and social contexts: Conceptualization, assessment and association with psychopathology. *Journal of Personality and Social Psychology, 60,* 456–70; Flett, G. L., & Hewitt, P. L. (2002). *Perfectionism: Theory, Research and Treatment.* American Psychological Association.

17 O'Connor, R. C., Rasmussen, S., & Hawton, K. (2010).Predicting depression, anxiety and self-harm in adolescents: The role of perfectionism and stress. *Behaviour Research and Therapy, 48,* 52–9.

18 Kahneman, D. (2011). *Thinking, Fast and Slow.* Penguin.

19 Greenwald, A. G., McGhee, D. E., & Schwartz, J. L. (1998). Measuring individual differences in implicit cognition: The implicit association test. *Journal of Personality and Social Psychology, 74,* 1464–80.

20 Nock, M. K., Park, J. M., Finn, C. T., Deliberto, T. L., Dour, H. J., & Banaji, M. R. (2010). Measuring the suicidal mind: Implicit cognition predicts suicidal behavior. *Psychological Science, 21,* 511–17.

21 Cha, C. B., O'Connor, R. C., Kirtley, O., Cleare, S., Wetherall, K., Eschle, S., Tezanos, K. M., & Nock, M. K. (2018). Testing mood-activated psychological markers for suicidal ideation. *Journal of Abnormal Psychology, 127,* 448–57.

22 Platt, S. (2016). Inequalities and suicidal behavior. In: O'Connor, R. C., & Pirkis, J. (eds.) (2016). *The International Handbook of Suicide Prevention.* Wiley-Blackwell, 258–83; Armstrong, G., Pirkis, J., Arabena, K., Currier, D., Spittal, M. J., & Jorm, A. F. (2017). Suicidal behaviour in Indigenous compared to non-Indigenous males in urban and regional Australia: Prevalence data suggest disparities increase across age groups. *Australian and New Zealand Journal of Psychiatry, 51,* 1240–8; Machado,

D. B., Rasella, D., & Dos Santos, D. N. (2015). Impact of income inequality and other social determinants on suicide rate in Brazil. *PLOS ONE, 10*, e0124934.

23 O'Connor, R. C., & Nock, M. K. (2014). The psychology of suicidal behaviour. *Lancet Psychiatry, 1*, 73–85; Chen, T., & Roberts, K. (2020). Negative life events and suicide in the national violent death reporting system. *Archives of Suicide Research.*

24 Turecki G. (2018) Early-life adversity and suicide risk: The role of epigenetics. In: Pompili M. (ed.) (2018). *Phenomenology of Suicide.* Springer.

25 Felitti, V. J., Anda, R. F., Nordenberg, D., Williamson, D. F., Spitz, A. M., Edwards, V., Koss, M. P., & Marks, J. S. (1998). Relationship of childhood abuse and household dysfunction to many of the leading causes of death in adults. The Adverse Childhood Experiences (ACE) Study. *American Journal of Preventive Medicine, 14*, 245–58; Bellis, M. A., Lowey, H., Leckenby, N., Hughes, K., & Harrison, D. (2014). Adverse childhood experiences: Retrospective study to determine their impact on adult health behaviours and health outcomes in a UK population. *Journal of Public Health, 36*, 81–91.

26 Dube, S. R., Anda, R. F., Felitti, V. J., Chapman, D. P., Williamson, D. F., & Giles, W. H. (2001). Childhood abuse, household dysfunction, and the risk of attempted suicide throughout the life span: findings from the Adverse Childhood Experiences Study. *JAMA, 286*, 3089–96.

27 Turecki G. (2018) Early-life adversity and suicide risk: The role of epigenetics. In: Pompili M. (ed.) (2018). *Phenomenology of Suicide.* Springer.

28 O'Connor, D. B., Gartland, N., & O'Connor, R. C. (2020). Stress, cortisol and suicide risk. *International Review of Neurobiology, 152*, 101–30.

29 O'Connor, D. B., Ferguson, E., Green, J., O'Carroll, R. E., & O'Connor, R. C. (2016). Cortisol levels and suicidal behavior: A

meta-analysis. *Psychoneuroendocrinology*, *63*, 370–9; Berardelli, I., Serafini, G., Cortese, N., Fiaschè, F., O'Connor, R. C., & Pompili, M. (2020). The involvement of hypothalamus-pituitary-adrenal (HPA) axis in suicide risk. *Brain Sciences*, *10*, 653; O'Connor, D. B., Branley-Bell, D., Green, J., Ferguson, E., Carroll, R. E., & O'Connor, R. C. (2020). Effects of childhood trauma, daily stress and emotions on daily cortisol levels in individuals vulnerable to suicide. *Journal of Abnormal Psychology*, *129*, 92–107.

30 O'Connor, D. B., & O'Connor, R. C. (9 Apr. 2020). Siblings. *The Psychologist*. Retrieved from https://thepsychologist.bps.org.uk/ siblings (accessed 1 Sep. 2020).

31 Smeets, T., Cornelisse, S., Quaedflieg, C. W. E. M., Meyer, T., Jelicic, M., & Merckelbach, H. (2012). Introducing the Maastricht Acute Stress Test (MAST): A quick and non-invasive approach to elicit robust autonomic and glucocorticoid stress responses. *Psychoneuroendocrinology*, *37*, 1998–2008.

32 O'Connor, D. B., Green, J. A., Ferguson, E., O'Carroll. R. E., & O'Connor, R. C. (2017). Cortisol reactivity and suicidal behavior: Investigating the role of the hypothalamic-pituitary-adrenal axis responses to stress in suicide attempters and ideators. *Psychoneuroendocrinology*, *75*, 183–91.

33 O'Connor, D. B., Green, J. A., Ferguson, E., O'Carroll, R. E., & O'Connor, R. C. (2018). Effects of childhood trauma on cortisol levels in suicide attempters and ideators. *Psychoneuroendocrinology*, *88*, 9–12.

34 O'Connor, D. B., Branley-Bell, D., Green, J. A., Ferguson, E., O'Carroll, R. E., & O'Connor, R. C. (2020). Effects of childhood trauma, daily stress, and emotions on daily cortisol levels in individuals vulnerable to suicide. *Journal of Abnormal Psychology*, *129*, 92–107.

35 Zortea, T. C., Gray, C. M., & O'Connor, R. C. (2019). The relationship between adult attachment and suicidal thoughts and behaviors: A systematic review. *Archives of Suicide Research*, *23*, 1–36.

36  Zortea, T. C., Dickson, A., Gray, C. M., O'Connor, R. C. (2019). Associations between experiences of disrupted attachments and suicidal thoughts and behaviours: An interpretative phenomenological analysis. *Social Science & Medicine, 235,* 112408.

37  van Orden, K., Witte, T. K., Cukrowicz, K. C., Braithwaite, S., Selby, E. A., Joiner, T. E. (2010). The interpersonal theory of suicide. *Psychological Review,* 117, 575–600.

38  Pollock, L. R., & Williams, J. M. (2001). Effective problem solving in suicide attempters depends on specific autobiographical recall. *Suicide & Life-Threatening Behavior, 31,* 386–96.

39  Pollock, L. R., & Williams, J. M. (2004). Problem-solving in suicide attempters. *Psychological Medicine, 34,* 163–7.

40  MacLeod, A. K., Pankhania, B., Lee, M., & Mitchell, D. (1997). Parasuicide, depression and the anticipation of positive and negative future experiences. *Psychological Medicine, 27,* 973–7.

41  MacLeod, A. K., & O'Connor, R. C. (2018). Positive future-thinking, wellbeing and mental health. In: Oettingen, G., Sevincer, A. T., & Gollwitzer, P. (eds.) (2018). *The Psychology of Thinking about the Future.* Guilford Publications Inc, 199–213.

42  O'Connor, R. C., Fraser, L., Whyte, M. C., Machale, S., & Masterton, G. (2008). A comparison of specific positive future expectancies and global hopelessness as predictors of suicidal ideation in a prospective study of repeat self-harmers. *Journal of Affective Disorders, 110,* 207–14.

43  O'Connor, R. C., Smyth, R., & Williams, J. M. G. (2015). Intrapersonal positive future thinking predicts repeat suicide attempts in hospital treated suicide attempters. *Journal of Consulting and Clinical Psychology, 83,* 169–76.

44  Cleare, S., Gumley, A., O'Connor, R. C. (2019). Self-compassion, forgiveness, suicidal ideation and self-harm: A systematic review. *Clinical Psychology & Psychotherapy, 26,* 511–30.

45  Cassidy, S., Bradley, P., Robinson, J., Allison, C., McHugh, M., & Baron-Cohen, S. (2014). Suicidal ideation and suicide plans or

attempts in adults with Asperger's syndrome attending a specialist diagnostic clinic: A clinical cohort study. *Lancet Psychiatry*, *1*, 142–7; Richards, G., Kenny, R., Griffiths, S., Allison, C., Mosse, D., Holt, R., O'Connor, R. C., Cassidy, S., & Baron-Cohen, S. (2019). Autistic traits in adults who have attempted suicide. *Molecular Autism*, *10*, 26.

46  Cassidy, S., & Rodgers, J. (2017). Understanding and prevention of suicide in autism. *Lancet Psychiatry*, *4*, e11.

47  Mak, J., Shires, D. A., Zhang, Q., . . . & Goodman, M. (2020). Suicide attempts among a cohort of transgender and gender diverse people. *American Journal of Preventive Medicine*, *59*, 570–7.

# Chapter 8: Crossing the Precipice: From Thoughts of Suicide to Suicidal Behaviour

1  Nock, M. K., Borges, G., Bromet, E. J., . . . & Williams, D. (2008). Cross-national prevalence and risk factors for suicidal ideation, plans and attempts. *British Journal of Psychiatry*, *192*, 98–105.

2  O'Connor, R. C., & Kirtley, O. J. (2018). The integrated motivational–volitional model of suicidal behaviour. *Philosophical Transactions of the Royal Society B.*, *373*, 20170268.

3  Ibid.

4  Norton, K. (20 Apr. 2018). Twitter. Retrieved from https://twitter.com/kennnaminh/status/987404512829861889 (accessed 3 Feb. 2021).

5  Zalsman, G., Hawton, K., Wasserman, D., van Heeringen, K., Arensman, E., Sarchiapone, M., Carli, V., Höschl, C., Barzilay, R., Balazs, J., Purebl, G., Kahn, J. P., Sáiz, P. A., Lipsicas, C. B., Bobes, J., Cozman, D., Hegerl, U., & Zohar, J. (2016). Suicide

prevention strategies revisited: 10-year systematic review. *Lancet Psychiatry*, 3, 646–59; Chen, Y-Y., Chien-Chang Wu, Wang, Y., & Yip, P. S. (2016). Suicide prevention through restricting access to suicide means and hotspots. In: O'Connor, R. C., & Pirkis, J. (eds.) (2016). *The International Handbook of Suicide Prevention*. Wiley-Blackwell, 609–36; Gunnell, D., Fernando, R., Hewagama, M., Priyangika, W. D., Konradsen, F., & Eddleston, M. (2007). The impact of pesticide regulations on suicide in Sri Lanka. *International Journal of Epidiololology*, 36, 1235–42.

6 Hawton, K. (2002). United Kingdom legislation on pack sizes of analgesics: Background, rationale, and effects on suicide and deliberate self-harm. *Suicide & Life-Threatening Behavior*, 32, 223–9.

7 Kreitman N. (1976). The coal gas story. United Kingdom suicide rates, 1960–71. *British Journal of Preventive & Social Medicine*, 30, 86–93.

8 Arya, V., Page, A., Gunnell, D., & Armstrong, G. (2021). Changes in method specific suicide following a national pesticide ban in India (2011–2014). *Journal of Affective Disorders*, 278, 592–600.

9 Mann, J. J., Apter, A., Bertolote, J., . . . & Hendin, H. (2005). Suicide prevention strategies: A systematic review. *JAMA*, 294, 2064–74.

10 Hawton, K. (2002). United Kingdom legislation on pack sizes of analgesics: Background, rationale, and effects on suicide and deliberate self-harm. *Suicide & Life-Threatening Behavior*, 32, 223–9; Hawton, K., Bergen, H., Simkin, S., Dodd, S., Pocock, P., Bernal, W., Gunnell, D., & Kapur, N. (2013). Long term effect of reduced pack sizes of paracetamol on poisoning deaths and liver transplant activity in England and Wales: Interrupted time series analyses. *BMJ*, 346, f403.

11 Pirkis, J., Too. L. S., Spittal, M. J., Krysinska, K., Robinson, J., Cheung, Y. T. (2015). Interventions to reduce suicides at suicide

hotspots: a systematic review and meta-analysis. *Lancet Psychiatry*, 2, 994–1001.

12  Gollwitzer, P. M., & Sheeran, P. (2006). Implementation intentions and goal achievement: A meta-analysis of effects and processes. In: Zanna, M. P. (ed.) (2006). *Advances in Experimental Social Psychology*. Elsevier Academic Press, vol. 38, 69–119.

13  Armitage, C. J., & Arden, M. A. (2012). A volitional help sheet to reduce alcohol consumption in the general population: a field experiment. *Prevention Science, 13*, 635–43; O'Connor, R. C., Ferguson, E., Scott, F., Smyth, R., McDaid, D., Park, A., Beautrais, A., & Armitage, C. J. (2017). A randomised controlled trial of a brief psychological intervention to reduce repetition of self-harm in patients admitted to hospital following a suicide attempt. *Lancet Psychiatry*, 4, 451–60.

14  Armitage, C. J., Abdul Rahim, W., Rowe, R. & O'Connor, R. C. (2016). An exploratory randomized trial of a simple, brief psychological intervention to reduce subsequent suicidal ideation and behaviour in patients hospitalised for self-harm. *British Journal of Psychiatry*, 208, 1–7.

15  O'Connor, R. C., Ferguson, E., Scott, F., Smyth, R., McDaid, D., Park, A., Beautrais, A., & Armitage, C. J. (2017). A randomised controlled trial of a brief psychological intervention to reduce repetition of self-harm in patients admitted to hospital following a suicide attempt. *Lancet Psychiatry*, 4, 451–60.

16  BBC Studios (2015). *Life After Suicide* [documentary]. Retrieved from https://www.bbc.co.uk/programmes/b05n2922 (accessed 21 Oct. 2020).

17  I wrote a blog about taking part in *Life After Suicide* for *The Psychologist*: O'Connor, R. (May 2015). Starting a national conversation about suicide. *The Psychologist*. Retrieved from https://thepsychologist.bps.org.uk/volume-28/may-2015/starting-national-conversation-about-suicide (accessed 20 Oct. 2020).

18  King, K., Schlichthorst, M., Keogh, L., Reifels, L., Spittal, M. J., Phelps, A., & Pirkis, J. (2019). Can watching a television documentary change the way men view masculinity? *Journal of Men's Studies*, 27, 287–306; King, K. E., Schlichthorst, M., Spittal, M. J., Phelps, A., & Pirkis, J. (2018). Can a documentary increase help-seeking intentions in men? A randomised controlled trial. *Journal of Epidemiology and Community Health*, 72, 92–8.

19  Erlangsen, A., & Pitman, A. (2017). Effects of suicide bereavement on mental and physical health. In: Andriessen, K., Krysinska, K., & Grad, O. T. (eds.) (2017). *Postvention in Action: The International Handbook of Suicide Bereavement Support*. Hogrefe Publishing, 17–26; Favril, L., O'Connor, R. C., Hawton, K., & Vander Laenen, F. (2020). Factors associated with the transition from suicidal ideation to suicide attempt in prison. *European Psychiatry*, 63, e101; Rostila, M., Saarela, J., & Kawachi, I. (2013). Suicide following the death of a sibling: A nationwide follow-up study from Sweden. *BMJ Open*, 3, e002618.

20  Pitman, A., Osborn, D., King, M., & Erlangsen, A. (2014). Effects of suicide bereavement on mental health and suicide risk. *Lancet Psychiatry*, 1, 86–94.

21  Garssen, J., Deerenberg, I., Mackenbach, J. P., Kerkhof, A., & Kunst, A. E. (2011). Familial risk of early suicide: Variations by age and sex of children and parents. *Suicide & Life-Threatening Behavior*, 41, 585–93.

22  Hua, P., Bugeja, L., & Maple, M. (2020). A systematic review on the relationship between childhood exposure to external cause parental death, including suicide, on subsequent suicidal behaviour. *Journal of Affective Disorders*, 257, 723–34.

23  Biddle, L., Gunnell, D., Owen-Smith, A., Potokar, J., Longson, D., Hawton, K., Kapur, N., & Donovan, J. (2012). Information sources used by the suicidal to inform choice of method. *Journal of Affective Disorders*, 136, 702–9; O'Connor, R. C., & Portzky,

G. (2018). Looking to the future: A synthesis of new developments and challenges in suicide research and prevention. *Frontiers in Psychology*, 9, 2139.

24 Turecki, G., & Brent, D. A. (2016). Suicide and suicidal behaviour. *Lancet*, 387(10024), 1227–39.

25 Netflix (2020). *The Social Dilemma* [documentary]. Retrieved from https://www.netflix.com/title/81254224 (accessed 3 Feb. 2021).

26 Ibid.

27 John, A., Glendenning, A. C., Marchant, A., Montgomery, P., Stewart, A., Wood, S., Lloyd, K., & Hawton, K. (2018). Self-harm, suicidal behaviours, and cyberbullying in children and young people: Systematic review. *Journal of Medical Internet Research*, 20, e129; Padmanathan, P., Bould, H., Winstone, L., Moran, P., & Gunnell, D. (2020). Social media use, economic recession and income inequality in relation to trends in youth suicide in high-income countries: A time trends analysis. *Journal of Affective Disorders*, 275, 58–65; O'Connor, R. C., & Robb, K. A. (2020). Identifying suicide risk factors in children is essential for developing effective prevention interventions. *Lancet Psychiatry*, 7, 292–3.

28 Reeves, A., McKee, M., & Stuckler, D. (2014). Economic suicides in the Great Recession in Europe and North America. *British Journal of Psychiatry*, 205, 246–7; Oyesanya, M., Lopez-Morinigo, J., & Dutta, R. (2015). Systematic review of suicide in economic recession. *World Journal of Psychiatry*, 5, 243–54.

29 Mojtabai, R., Olfson, M., & Han, B. (2016). National trends in the prevalence and treatment of depression in adolescents and young adults. *Pediatrics*, 138, e20161878.

30 Robinson, J., Cox, G., Bailey, E., Hetrick, S., Rodrigues, M., Fisher, S., & Herrman, H. (2016). Social media and suicide prevention: A systematic review. *Early Intervention in Psychiatry*, 10, 103–21;

Marchant, A., Hawton, K., Stewart, A., Montgomery, P., Singaravelu, V., Lloyd, K., Purdy, N., Daine, K., & John, A. (2017). A systematic review of the relationship between internet use, self-harm and suicidal behaviour in young people: The good, the bad and the unknown. *PLOS ONE, 12,* e0181722.

31 Biernesser, C., Sewall, C., Brent, D., Bear, T., Mair, C., & Trauth, J. (2020). Social media use and deliberate self-harm among youth: A systematized narrative review. *Children and Youth Services Review, 116,* 105054.

32 John, A., Glendenning, A. C., Marchant, A., Montgomery, P., Stewart, A., Wood, S., Lloyd, K., & Hawton, K. (2018). Self-harm, suicidal behaviours, and cyberbullying in children and young people: Systematic review. *Journal of Medical Internet Research, 20,* e129.

33 Hawton, K., Simkin, S., Deeks, J. J., O'Connor, S., Keen, A., Altman, D. G., Philo, G., & Bulstrode, C. (1999). Effects of a drug overdose in a television drama on presentations to hospital for self poisoning: Time series and questionnaire study. *BMJ, 318*(7189), 972–7.

34 Netflix (2017). *13 Reasons Why.* Retrieved from https://www.netflix.com/title/80117470 (accessed 3 Feb. 2021).

35 World Health Organization/International Association for Suicide Prevention (2017). Media guidelines. Retrieved from https://www.iasp.info/media_guidelines.php (accessed 9 Jan. 2021).

36 O'Connor, R. (2 May 2017). Comment on the Netflix series 13 Reasons Why [blog]. Suicidal Behaviour Research Lab. Retrieved from http://www.suicideresearch.info/news-1/commentonthenetflixseries13reasonswhy (accessed 11 Jan. 2021).

37 Niederkrotenthaler, T., Stack, S., Till, B., Sinyor, M., Pirkis, J., Garcia, D., Rockett, I., & Tran, U. S. (2019). Association of increased youth suicides in the United States with the release of *13 Reasons Why. JAMA Psychiatry, 76,* 933–40.

38 Bridge, J. A., Greenhouse, J. B., Ruch, D., Stevens, J., Ackerman, J., Sheftall, A. H., Horowitz, L. M., Kelleher, K. J., & Campo,

J. V. (2020). Association between the release of Netflix's *13 Reasons Why* and suicide rates in the United States: An interrupted time series analysis. *Journal of the American Academy of Child and Adolescent Psychiatry*, *59*, 236–43.

39 Romer, D. (2020). Reanalysis of the Bridge et al. study of suicide following release of *13 Reasons Why*. *PLOS ONE*, *15*, e0227545; Bridge, J. A., Greenhouse, J. B., Kelleher, K. J., & Campo, J. V. (2020). Formal comment: Romer study fails at following core principles of reanalysis. *PLOS ONE*, *15*, e0237184.

40 Karter, E. (22 Mar. 2018). Multinational study: How teens, parents respond to Netflix show '13 Reasons Why'. Northwestern University. Retrieved from https://news.northwestern.edu/stories/2018/march/13-reasons-why/ (accessed 5 Jan. 2021).

41 Niederkrotenthaler, T., Fu, K. W., Yip, P. S., Fong, D. Y., Stack, S., Cheng, Q., & Pirkis, J. (2012). Changes in suicide rates following media reports on celebrity suicide: A meta-analysis. *Journal of Epidemiology and Community Health*, *66*, 1037–42.

42 Phillips D. P. (1974). The influence of suggestion on suicide: Substantive and theoretical implications of the Werther effect. *American Sociological Review*, *39*, 340–54.

43 Niederkrotenthaler, T., Braun, M., Pirkis, J., Till, B., Stack, S., Sinyor, M., Tran, U. S., Voracek, M., Cheng, Q., Arendt, F., Scherr, S., Yip, P., & Spittal, M. J. (2020). Association between suicide reporting in the media and suicide: Systematic review and meta-analysis. *BMJ*, *368*, m575.

44 Niederkrotenthaler, T., Voracek, M., Herberth, A., Till, B., Strauss, M., Etzersdorfer, E., Eisenwort, B., & Sonneck, G. (2010). Role of media reports in completed and prevented suicide: Werther v. Papageno effects. *British Journal of Psychiatry*, *197*, 234–43.

45 Robinson, J., Pirkis, J., & O'Connor, R. C. (2016). Suicide clusters. In: O'Connor, R. C., & Pirkis, J. (eds.) (2016). *The International Handbook of Suicide Prevention*. Wiley-Blackwell, 758–74.

46  Joiner, T. E. (2003). Contagion of suicidal symptoms as a function of assortative relating and shared relationship stress in college roommates. *Journal of Adolescence, 26,* 495–504.

47  Gvion, Y., & Apter, A. (2011). Aggression, impulsivity, and suicide behavior: A review of the literature. *Archives of Suicide Research, 15,* 93–112; Anestis, M. D., Soberay, K. A., Gutierrez, P. M., Hernandez, T. D., & Joiner, T. E. (2014). Reconsidering the link between impulsivity and suicidal behavior. *Personality and Social Psychology Review, 18,* 366–86; McHugh, C. M., Lee, R. S. C., Hermens, D. F., Corderoy, A., Large, M., & Hickie, I. B. (2019). Impulsivity in the self-harm and suicidal behavior of young people: A systematic review and meta-analysis. *Journal of Psychiatric Research, 116,* 51–60.

48  Wetherall, K., Cleare, S., Eschle, S., Ferguson, E., O'Connor, D. B., O'Carroll, R., & O'Connor, R. C. (2018). From ideation to action: Differentiating between those who think about suicide and those who attempt suicide in a national study of young adults. *Journal of Affective Disorders, 241,* 475–83; Branley-Bell, D., O'Connor, D. B., Green, J. A., Ferguson, E., O'Carroll, R. E., & O'Connor, R. C. (2019). Distinguishing suicide ideation from suicide attempts: Further test of the integrated motivational–volitional model of suicidal behaviour. *Journal of Psychiatric Research, 117,* 100–7; Dhingra, K., Boduszek, D., & O'Connor, R. C. (2015). Differentiating suicide attempters from suicide ideators using the integrated motivational–volitional model of suicidal behaviour. *Journal of Affective Disorders, 186,* 211–8.

49  Millner, A. J., Lee, M. D., Hoyt, K., Buckholtz, J. W., Auerbach, R. P., & Nock, M. K. (2020). Are suicide attempters more impulsive than suicide ideators? *General Hospital Psychiatry, 63,* 103–10; Anestis, M. D., & Joiner, T. E. (2011). Examining the role of emotion in suicidality: Negative urgency as an amplifier of the relationship between components of the

interpersonal-psychological theory of suicidal behavior and lifetime number of suicide attempts. *Journal of Affective Disorders*, *129*, 261–9.

50 Melson, A. J., & O'Connor, R. C. (2019). Differentiating adults who think about self-harm from those who engage in self-harm: The role of volitional alcohol factors. *BMC Psychiatry*, *19*, 319.

51 Smith, P. N., Stanley, I. H., Joiner, T. E., Jr, Sachs-Ericsson, N. J., & Van Orden, K. A. (2016). An aspect of the capability for suicide-fearlessness of the pain involved in dying-amplifies the association between suicide ideation and attempts. *Archives of Suicide Research*, *20*, 650–62.

52 Klonsky, E. D., & May, A. M. (2015). The three-step theory (3ST): A new theory of suicide rooted in the 'ideation-to-action' framework. *International Journal of Cognitive Therapy*, *8*, 114–29.

53 Klonsky, E. D., Saffer, B. Y., & Bryan, C. J. (2018). Ideation-to-action theories of suicide: A conceptual and empirical update. *Current Opinion in Psychology*, *22*, 38–43.

54 Chu, C., Buchman-Schmitt, J. M., Stanley, I. H., Hom, M. A., Tucker, R. P., Hagan, C. R., Rogers, M. L., Podlogar, M. C., Chiurliza, B., Ringer, F. B., Michaels, M. S., Patros, C., & Joiner, T. E. (2017). The interpersonal theory of suicide: A systematic review and meta-analysis of a decade of cross-national research. *Psychological Bulletin*, *143*, 1313–45.

55 Kirtley, O. J., O'Carroll, R. E., & O'Connor, R. C. (2015). Hurting inside and out? Emotional and physical pain in self-harm ideation and enactment. *International Journal of Cognitive Therapy*, *8*, 156–71; Osman, A., Barrios, F. X., Gutierrez, P. M., Schwarting, B., Kopper, B. A., & Mei-ChuanWang (2005). Reliability and construct validity of the pain distress inventory. *Journal of Behavioral Medicine*, *28*, 169–80; Kirtley, O. J., O'Carroll, R. E., & O'Connor, R. C. (2015). The role of endogenous opioids in non-suicidal self-injurious behavior: Methodological Challenges. *Neuroscience & Biobehavioral Review*, *48*, 186–9.

56 Law, K. C., Khazem, L. R., Jin, H. M., & Anestis, M. D. (2017). Non-suicidal self-injury and frequency of suicide attempts: The role of pain persistence. *Journal of Affective Disorders, 209,* 254–61.

57 Kirtley, O. J., O'Carroll, R. E., & O'Connor, R. C. (2016). Pain and self-harm: A systematic review. *Journal of Affective Disorders, 203,* 347–63.

58 Kirtley, O. J., Rodham, K., & Crane, C. (2020). Understanding suicidal ideation and behaviour in individuals with chronic pain: A review of the role of novel transdiagnostic psychological factors. *Lancet Psychiatry, 7,* 282–90.

59 Freud, S. (1922). *Beyond the Pleasure Principle.* Bartleby.com, Hubback, C. J. M. (trans.).

60 Menninger, K. (1938). *Man Against Himself.* Mariner Books.

61 Chu, C., Buchman-Schmitt, J. M., Stanley, I. H., Hom, M. A., Tucker, R. P., Hagan, C. R., Rogers, M. L., Podlogar, M. C., Chiurliza, B., Ringer, F. B., Michaels, M. S., Patros, C., & Joiner, T. E. (2017). The interpersonal theory of suicide: A systematic review and meta-analysis of a decade of cross-national research. *Psychological Bulletin, 143,* 1313–45.

62 Ribeiro, J. D., Witte, T. K., van Orden, K. A., Selby, E. A., Gordon, K. H., Bender, T. W., & Joiner, T. E. (2014). Fearlessness about death: The psychometric properties and construct validity of the revision to the acquired capability for suicide scale. *Psychological Assessment, 26,* 115–26.

63 Wetherall, K., Cleare, S., Eschle, S., Ferguson, E., O'Connor, D. B., O'Carroll, R. E., & O'Connor, R. C. (2018). From ideation to action: differentiating between those who think about suicide and those who attempt suicide in a national study of young adults. *Journal of Affective Disorders, 241,* 475–83.

64 McCormick, A., Meijen, C., & Marcora, S. (2015). Psychological determinants of whole-body endurance performance. *Sports Medicine, 45,* 997–1015.

65 Wetherall, K., Cleare, S., Eschle, S., Ferguson, E., O'Connor, D. B., O'Carroll, R. E., & O'Connor, R. C. (2018). From ideation to action: Differentiating between those who think about suicide and those who attempt suicide in a national study of young adults. *Journal of Affective Disorders*, 241, 475–83.

66 Holmes, E. A., Crane, C., Fennell, M. J., & Williams, J. M. (2007). Imagery about suicide in depression – 'Flash-forwards'? *Journal of Behavior Therapy and Experimental Psychiatry*, 38, 423–34; Crane, C., Shah, D., Barnhofer, T., & Holmes, E. A. (2012). Suicidal imagery in a previously depressed community sample. *Clinical Psychology & Psychotherapy*, 19, 57–69.

67 Naherniak, B., Bhaskaran, J., Sareen, J., Wang, Y., & Bolton, J. M. (2019). Ambivalence about living and the risk for future suicide attempts: A longitudinal analysis. *The Primary Care Companion for CNS Disorders*, 21, 18m02361.

68 Ng, R., Di Simplicio, M., McManus, F., Kennerley, H., & Holmes, E.A. (2016). 'Flash-forwards' and suicidal ideation: A prospective investigation of mental imagery, entrapment and defeat in a cohort from the Hong Kong Mental Morbidity Survey. *Psychiatry Research*, 246, 453–60.

69 Di Simplicio, M., Appiah-Kusi, E., Wilkinson, P., Watson, P., Meiser-Stedman, C., Kavanagh, D. J., & Holmes, E. A. (2020). Imaginator: A proof-of-concept feasibility trial of a brief imagery-based psychological intervention for young people who self-harm. *Suicide & Life-Threatening Behavior*, 50, 724–40.

70 Chan, M. K., Bhatti, H., Meader, N., Stockton, S., Evans, J., O'Connor, R. C., Kapur, N., & Kendall, T. (2016). Predicting suicide following self-harm: Systematic review of risk factors and risk scales. *British Journal of Psychiatry*, 209, 277–83; Mars, B., Heron, J., Klonsky, E. D., Moran, P., O'Connor, R. C., Tilling, K., Wilkinson, P., & Gunnell, D. (2019). Predictors of future suicide attempt among adolescents with suicidal thoughts or non-suicidal self-harm: A birth cohort study. *Lancet Psychiatry*,

6, 327–37; Favril, L., & O'Connor, R. C. (2019). Distinguishing prisoners who think about suicide from those who attempt suicide. *Psychological Medicine*, 1–8.

71 Franklin, J. C., Ribeiro, J. D., Fox, K. R., Bentley, K. H., Kleiman, E. M., Huang, X., Musacchio, K. M., Jaroszewski, A. C., Chang, B. P., & Nock, M. K. (2017). Risk factors for suicidal thoughts and behaviors: A meta-analysis of 50 years of research. *Psychological Bulletin*, *143*, 187–232.

72 Cooper, J., Kapur, N., Webb, R., Lawlor, M., Guthrie, E., Mackway-Jones, K., & Appleby, L. (2005). Suicide after deliberate self-harm: A 4-year cohort study. *American Journal of Psychiatry*, *162*, 297–303.

73 O'Connor, R. C., Ferguson, E., Scott, F., Smyth, R., McDaid, D., Park, A., Beautrais, A., & Armitage, C. J. (2017). A randomised controlled trial of a brief psychological intervention to reduce repetition of self-harm in patients admitted to hospital following a suicide attempt. *Lancet Psychiatry*, *4*, 451–60; O'Connor, R. C., Smyth, R., Ferguson, E., Ryan, C., & Williams, J. M. G. (2013). Psychological processes and repeat suicidal behavior: A four year prospective study. *Journal of Consulting & Clinical Psychology*, *81*, 1137–43.

74 Carroll, R., Metcalfe, C., & Gunnell, D. (2014). Hospital management of self-harm patients and risk of repetition: Systematic review and meta-analysis. *Journal of Affective Disorders*, *168*, 476–83.

75 O'Connor, R. C., & Kirtley, O. J. (2018). The integrated motivational–volitional model of suicidal behaviour. *Philosophical Transactions of the Royal Society B.*, *373*, 20170268.

76 Jordan, J. T., & McNiel, D. E. (2020). Characteristics of persons who die on their first suicide attempt: Results from the National Violent Death Reporting System. *Psychological Medicine*, *50*, 1390–7; O'Connor, R. C., & Sheehy, N. P (1997). Suicide and gender. *Mortality*, *2*, 239–54.

77  Townsend, E., Wadman, R., Sayal, K., Armstrong, M., Harroe, C., Majumder, P., Vostanis, P., & Clarke, D. (2016). Uncovering key patterns in self-harm in adolescents: Sequence analysis using the Card Sort Task for Self-harm (CaTS). *Journal of Affective Disorders*, *206*, 161–8.

78  Samaritans (n.d.). Middle-aged men and suicide. Retrieved from https://www.samaritans.org/scotland/about-samaritans/research-policy/middle-aged-men-suicide (accessed 2 Feb. 2021).

79  O'Connor, R. C., & Noyce, R. (2008). Personality and cognitive processes: Self-criticism and different types of rumination as predictors of suicidal ideation. *Behaviour Research and Therapy*, *46*, 392–401.

80  Morrison, R., & O'Connor, R. C. (2008). A systematic review of the relationship between rumination and suicidality. *Suicide and Life-Threatening Behavior*, *38*, 523–38.

81  Thompson, M. P., Kingree, J. B., & Lamis, D. (2019). Associations of adverse childhood experiences and suicidal behaviors in adulthood in a U.S. nationally representative sample. *Child: Care, Health and Development*, *45*, 121–8.

82  Wyllie, C., Platt, S., Brownlie, J., Chandler, A., Connolly, S., Evans, R., Kennelly, B., Kirtley, O., Moore, G., O'Connor, R., & Scourfield, J. (2012). Men, suicide and society. Why disadvantaged men in mid-life die by suicide. Samaritans. Retrieved from https://media.samaritans.org/documents/Samaritans_MenSuicideSociety_ResearchReport2012.pdf (accessed 27 Jan. 2021).

## Chapter 9: Brief Contact Interventions

1  O'Connor, R. C., Ferguson, E., Scott, F., Smyth, R., McDaid, D., Park, A., Beautrais, A., & Armitage, C. J. (2017). A randomised controlled trial of a brief psychological intervention to reduce

repetition of self-harm in patients admitted to hospital following a suicide attempt. *Lancet Psychiatry*, 4, 451–60; Gollwitzer, P. M., & Sheeran, P. (2006). Implementation intentions and goal achievement: A meta-analysis of effects and processes. In: Zanna, M. P. (ed.) (2006), *Advances in Experimental Social Psychology*. Elsevier Academic Press, vol. 38, 69–119.

2 O'Connor, R. C., & Kirtley, O. J. (2018). The integrated motivational–volitional model of suicidal behaviour. *Philosophical Transactions of the Royal Society B.*, 373, 20170268; van Orden, K., Witte, T. K., Cukrowicz, K. C., Braithwaite, S., Selby, E. A., & Joiner, T. E. (2010). The interpersonal theory of suicide. *Psychological Review*, 117, 575–600; Sheehy, K., Noureen, A., Khaliq, A., Dhingra, K., Husain, N., Pontin, E. E., Cawley, R., & Taylor, P. J. (2019). An examination of the relationship between shame, guilt and self-harm: A systematic review and meta-analysis. *Clinical Psychology Review*, 73, 101779.

3 Saunders, K. E., Hawton, K., Fortune, S., & Farrell, S. (2012). Attitudes and knowledge of clinical staff regarding people who self-harm: A systematic review. *Journal of Affective Disorders*, 139, 205–16; Taylor, T. L., Hawton, K., Fortune, S., & Kapur, N. (2009). Attitudes towards clinical services among people who self-harm: Systematic review. *British Journal of Psychiatry*, 194, 104–10.

4 Motto, J. A., & Bostrom, A. G. (2001). A randomized controlled trial of postcrisis suicide prevention. *Psychiatric Services*, 52, 828–33.

5 Ibid.

6 Ibid.

7 Milner, A. J., Carter, G., Pirkis, J., Robinson, J., & Spittal, M. J. (2015). Letters, green cards, telephone calls and postcards: Systematic and meta-analytic review of brief contact interventions for reducing self-harm, suicide attempts and suicide. *British Journal of Psychiatry*, 206, 184–90; Hetrick, S. E., Robinson, J., Spittal, M. J., & Carter, G. (2016). Effective psychological and

psychosocial approaches to reduce repetition of self-harm: A systematic review, meta-analysis and meta-regression. *BMJ Open*, *6*, e011024; Hawton, K., Witt, K. G., Salisbury, T., Arensman, E., Gunnell, D., Hazell, P., Townsend, E., & van Heeringen, K. (2016). Psychosocial interventions following self-harm in adults: A systematic review and meta-analysis. *Lancet Psychiatry*, *3*, 740–50.

8 Milner, A. J., Carter, G., Pirkis, J., Robinson, J., & Spittal, M. J. (2015). Letters, green cards, telephone calls and postcards: Systematic and meta-analytic review of brief contact interventions for reducing self-harm, suicide attempts and suicide. *British Journal of Psychiatry*, *206*, 184–90.

9 O'Connor, R. C., Ferguson, E., Scott, F., Smyth, R., McDaid, D., Park, A., Beautrais, A., & Armitage, C. J. (2017). A randomised controlled trial of a brief psychological intervention to reduce repetition of self-harm in patients admitted to hospital following a suicide attempt. *Lancet Psychiatry*, *4*, 451–60.

# Chapter 10: Safety Planning

1 Doupnik, S. K., Rudd, B., Schmutte, T., Worsley, D., Bowden, C. F., McCarthy, E., Eggan, E., Bridge, J. A., & Marcus, S. C. (2020). Association of Suicide Prevention interventions with subsequent suicide attempts, linkage to follow-up care, and depression symptoms for acute care settings: A systematic review and meta-analysis. *JAMA Psychiatry*, *77*, 1021–30.

2 Suicide Prevention Resource Center. Provides useful resources for training in suicide prevention: https://www.sprc.org.

3 Stanley, B., & Brown, G. K. (2012). Safety planning intervention: A brief intervention to mitigate suicide risk. *Cognitive & Behavioral Practice*, *19*, 256–64.

4 Ibid.

5 O'Connor, R. C., Ferguson, E., Scott, F., Smyth, R., McDaid, D., Park, A., Beautrais, A., & Armitage, C. J. (2017). A randomised controlled trial of a brief psychological intervention to reduce repetition of self-harm in patients admitted to hospital following a suicide attempt. *Lancet Psychiatry*, 4, 451–60.

6 Stanley, B., Brown, G. K., Brenner, L. A., Galfalvy, H. C., Currier, G. W., Knox, K. L., Chaudhury, S. R., Bush, A. L., & Green, K. L. (2018). Comparison of the safety planning intervention with follow-up vs usual care of suicidal patients treated in the emergency department. *JAMA Psychiatry*, 75, 894–900; Stanley, B., Chaudhury, S. R., Chesin, M., Pontoski, K., Bush, A. M., Knox, K. L., & Brown, G. K. (2016). An emergency department intervention and follow-up to reduce suicide risk in the VA: Acceptability and effectiveness. *Psychiatric Services*, 67, 680–3; Doupnik, S. K., Rudd, B., Schmutte, T., Worsley, D., Bowden, C. F., McCarthy, E., Eggan, E., Bridge, J. A., & Marcus, S. C. (2020). Association of Suicide Prevention interventions with subsequent suicide attempts, linkage to follow-up care, and depression symptoms for acute care settings: A systematic review and meta-analysis. *JAMA Psychiatry*, 77, 1021–30.

7 Stanley, B., Brown, G. K., Brenner, L. A., Galfalvy, H. C., Currier, G. W., Knox, K. L., Chaudhury, S. R., Bush, A. L., & Green, K. L. (2018). Comparison of the safety planning intervention with follow-up vs usual care of suicidal patients treated in the emergency department. *JAMA Psychiatry*, 75, 894–900.

8 O'Connor, R. C., Lundy, J-M., Stewart, C., Smillie, S., McClelland, H., Syrett, S., Gavigan, M., McConnachie, A., Smith, M., Smith, D. J., Brown, G., Stanley B., & Simpson, S. A. (2019). Study protocol for the SAFETEL randomised controlled feasibility trial of a safety planning intervention with follow-up telephone contact to reduce suicidal behaviour. *BMJ Open*, 9(2).

9 Stanley, B., & Brown, G. K. (2017). *Safety Planning Intervention Manual.* Unpublished.

10 Bryan, C. J., Rozek, D. C., Butner, J., & Rudd, M. D. (2019). Patterns of change in suicide ideation signal the recurrence of suicide attempts among high-risk psychiatric outpatients. *Behaviour Research and Therapy, 120,* 103392.

11 Kleiman, E. M., & Nock, M. K. (2018). Real-time assessment of suicidal thoughts and behaviors. *Current Opinion in Psychology, 22,* 33–7.

12 Health Education England (HEE), & National Collaborating Centre for Mental Health (NCCMH) (n.d.). Self-harm and suicide prevention competency frameworks. Retrieved from https://www.hee.nhs.uk/our-work/mental-health/self-harm-suicide-prevention-frameworks (accessed 27 Jan. 2021).

13 Rodgers, J., Kasim, A., Heslop, P., Cassidy, S., Ramsay, S., Wilson, C., Townsend, E., Vale, L., & O'Connor, R. C. (Sep. 2020). Adapted suicide safety plans to address self harm, suicidal ideation and suicide behaviours in autistic adults: An interventional single arm feasibility trial and external pilot randomised controlled trial [ongoing research study funded by National Institute of Health Research]. Retrieved from https://fundingawards.nihr.ac.uk/award/NIHR129196 (accessed 9 Dec. 2020).

14 Stanley, B., & Brown, G. K. (2012). Safety planning intervention: A brief intervention to mitigate suicide risk. *Cognitive & Behavioral Practice, 19,* 256–64; Stanley, B., & Brown, G.K. (2017). *Safety Planning Intervention Manual.* Unpublished; O'Connor, R. C., Lundy, J. M., Stewart, C., Smillie, S., McClelland, H., Syrett, S., Gavigan, M., McConnachie, A., Smith, M., Smith, D. J., Brown, G. K., Stanley, B., & Simpson, S. A. (2019). SAFETEL randomised controlled feasibility trial of a safety planning intervention with follow-up telephone contact to reduce suicidal behaviour: Study protocol. *BMJ Open, 9,* e025591.

15 Miller, W. R., & Rollnick, S. (2013). *Motivational Interviewing: Helping People Change.* Guilford Press, third edition.

16 Stanley, B., Martínez-Alés, G., Gratch, I., Rizk, M., Galfalvy, H., Choo, T. H., & Mann, J. J. (2021). Coping strategies that reduce suicidal ideation: An ecological momentary assessment study. *Journal of Psychiatric Research*, *133*, 32–7.

17 de Beurs, D., Kirtley, O., Kerkhof, A., Portzky, G., & O'Connor, R. C. (2015). The role of mobile phone technology in understanding and preventing suicidal behavior. *Crisis*, *36*, 79–82; Nuij, C., van Ballegooijen, W., Ruwaard, J., de Beurs, D., Mokkenstorm, J., van Duijn, E., de Winter, R., O'Connor, R. C., Smit, J. H., Riper, H., & Kerkhof, A. (2018). Smartphone-based safety planning and self-monitoring for suicidal patients: Rationale and study protocol of the CASPAR (Continuous Assessment for Suicide Prevention And Research) study. *Internet Interventions*, *13*, 16–23.

18 Stanley, I. H., Hom, M. A., Rogers, M. L., Anestis, M. D., & Joiner, T. E. (2017). Discussing firearm ownership and access as part of suicide risk assessment and prevention: 'Means safety' versus 'means restriction'. *Archives of Suicide Research*, *21*, 237–53; Anestis, M. D. (2018). *Guns and Suicide: An American Epidemic.* Oxford University Press.

19 Brown, G. K., & Stanley, B. (2017). *Safety Plan Pocket Card.* Unpublished.

## Chapter 11: Longer-Term Interventions

1 Hawton, K., Witt, K. G., Taylor Salisbury, T. L., Arensman, E., Gunnell, D., Hazell, P., Townsend, E., & van Heeringen, K. (2016). Psychosocial interventions for self-harm in adults. *Cochrane Database of Systematic Reviews*, (5), CD012189; Hawton, K., Witt,

K. G., Taylor Salisbury, T. L., Arensman, E., Gunnell, D., Townsend, E., van Heeringen, K., & Hazell, P. (2015). Interventions for self-harm in children and adolescents. *Cochrane Database of Systematic Reviews*, (12), CD012013.

2 MQ Transforming Mental Health (Apr. 2015). UK mental health research funding. Retrieved from https://b.3cdn.net/joinmq/1f731755e4183d5337_apm6b0gll.pdf (accessed 20 Nov. 2020).

3 Carey, B. (23 Jun. 2011). Expert on mental illness reveals her own fight. *New York Times*. Retrieved from http://archive.nytimes.com/www.nytimes.com/2011/06/23/health/23lives.html (accessed 31 Jan. 2021).

4 Linehan, M. M., Comtois, K. A., Murray, A. M., Brown, M. Z., Gallop, R. J., Heard, H. L., Korslund, K. E., Tutek, D. A., Reynolds, S. K., & Lindenboim, N. (2006). Two-year randomized controlled trial and follow-up of dialectical behavior therapy vs therapy by experts for suicidal behaviors and borderline personality disorder. *Archives of General Psychiatry*, *63*, 757–66.

5 Mehlum, L., Tørmoen, A. J., Ramberg, M., Haga, E., Diep, L. M., Laberg, S., Larsson, B. S., Stanley, B. H., Miller, A. L., Sund, A. M., & Grøholt, B. (2014). Dialectical behavior therapy for adolescents with repeated suicidal and self-harming behavior: A randomized trial. *Journal of the American Academy of Child and Adolescent Psychiatry*, *53*, 1082–91.

6 Beck, A., Rush, A. J., Shaw, B. E., & Emery, G. (1987). *Cognitive Therapy for Depression*. Guildford Press.

7 Information and resources for CBT are available via the Beck Institute: https://beckinstitute.org.

8 Brown, G. K., Ten Have, T., Henriques, G. R., Xie, S. X., Hollander, J. E., & Beck, A. T. (2005). Cognitive therapy for the prevention of suicide attempts: A randomized controlled trial. *JAMA*, *294*, 563–70.

9 Rudd, M. D., Bryan, C. J., Wertenberger, E. G., Peterson, A. L., Young-McCaughan, S., Mintz, J., Williams, S. R., Arne, K. A., Breitbach, J., Delano, K., Wilkinson, E., & Bruce, T. O. (2015). Brief cognitive-behavioral therapy effects on post-treatment suicide attempts in a military sample: Results of a randomized clinical trial with 2-year follow-up. *American Journal of Psychiatry*, *172*, 441–9.

10 Rossouw, T. I., & Fonagy, P. (2012). Mentalization-based treatment for self-harm in adolescents: A randomized controlled trial. *Journal of the American Academy of Child and Adolescent Psychiatry*, *51*, 1304–13.e3.

11 Ougrin, D., Tranah, T., Stahl, D., Moran, P., & Asarnow, J. R. (2015). Therapeutic interventions for suicide attempts and self-harm in adolescents: Systematic review and meta-analysis. *Journal of the American Academy of Child and Adolescent Psychiatry*, *54*, 97–107.e2.

12 Jobes, D. A. (2016). *Managing Suicide Risk: A Collaborative Approach*. Guilford Press.

13 Jobes, D. A. (2012). The Collaborative Assessment and Management of Suicidality (CAMS): An evolving evidence-based clinical approach to suicidal risk. *Suicide & Life-Threatening Behavior*, *42*, 640–53; Comtois, K. A., Jobes, D. A., O'Connor, S., Atkins, D. C., Janis, K., Chessen, C., Landes, S. J., Holen, A., & Yuodelis Flores, C. (2011). Collaborative Assessment and Management of Suicidality (CAMS): Feasibility trial for next-day appointment services. *Depression and Anxiety*, *28*, 963–72.

14 A list of all of the research studies for CAMS is available at: CAMS-Care Preventing Suicide. Retrieved from https://cams-care.com/about-cams/the-evidence-base-for-cams (accessed 27 Jan. 2021).

15 Gysin-Maillart, A., Schwab, S., Soravia, L., Megert, M., & Michel, K. (2016). A novel brief therapy for patients who attempt suicide: A 24-months follow-up randomized controlled study of the

Attempted Suicide Short Intervention Program (ASSIP). *PLOS Medicine*, *13*, e1001968.

16 The Aeschi Working Group: http://www.aeschiconference.unibe. ch (accessed 30 Jan. 2021).

17 Attempted Suicide Short Intervention Program (ASSIP): https://www.assip.ch (accessed 27 Jan. 2021).

18 Gysin-Maillart, A., Schwab, S., Soravia, L., Megert, M., & Michel, K. (2016). A novel brief therapy for patients who attempt suicide: A 24-months follow-up randomized controlled study of the Attempted Suicide Short Intervention Program (ASSIP). *PLOS Medicine*, *13*, e1001968.

19 National Confidential Inquiry into Suicide and Safety in Mental Health (Dec. 2019). Annual report 2019: England, Northern Ireland, Scotland and Wales. Retrieved from https://sites.manchester. ac.uk/ncish/reports/annual-report-2019-england-northern-ireland-scotland-and-wales/ (accessed 9 July. 2020).

20 Perry, Y., Werner-Seidler, A., Calear, A. L., & Christensen, H. (2016). Web-based and mobile suicide prevention interventions for young people: A systematic review. *Journal of the Canadian Academy of Child and Adolescent Psychiatry*, *25*, 73–9.

21 Torok, M., Han, J., Baker, S., Werner-Seidler, A., Wong, I., Larsen, M.E., & Christensen, H. (2020). Suicide prevention using self-guided digital interventions: A systematic review and meta-analysis of randomised controlled trials. *Lancet Digital Health*, *2*, e25–36; Tighe, J., Shand, F., Ridani, R., Mackinnon, A., De La Mata, N., & Christensen, H. (2017). Ibobbly mobile health intervention for suicide prevention in Australian Indigenous youth: A pilot randomised controlled trial. *BMJ Open*, *7*, e013518.

22 Stapelberg, N., Sveticic, J., Hughes, I., Almeida-Crasto, A., Gaee-Atefi, T., Gill, N., ... & Turner, K. (2020). Efficacy of the Zero Suicide framework in reducing recurrent suicide attempts: Cross-sectional and time-to-recurrent-event analyses. *British Journal of*

*Psychiatry*, 1–10; Zortea, T. C., Cleare, S., Melson, A. J., Wetherall, K., & O'Connor, R. C. (2020). Understanding and managing suicide risk. *British Medical Bulletin*, *134*, 73–84.

# Chapter 12: Asking People About Suicide

1 BBC Three (2015). *Suicide and Me* [documentary]. Retrieved from https://www.bbc.co.uk/programmes/b06mvx4j (accessed 21 Nov. 2020).

2 United to Prevent Suicide: https://unitedtopreventsuicide.org.uk (accessed 22 Nov. 2020).

3 Samaritans (n.d.). Small Talk Saves Lives. Retrieved from https://www.samaritans.org/support-us/campaign/small-talk-saves-lives (accessed 22 Nov. 2020).

4 Marzano, L., Mackenzie, J. M., Kruger, I., Borrill, J., & Fields, B. (2019). Factors deterring and prompting the decision to attempt suicide on the railway networks: Findings from 353 online surveys and 34 semi-structured interviews. *British Journal of Psychiatry*, 1–6.

5 R U OK? (9 Sep. 2019). Working together to prevent suicide. Retrieved from https://www.ruok.org.au/working-together-to-prevent-suicide (accessed 22 Nov. 2020).

6 Platt, S., McLean, J., McCollam, A., Blamey, A., Mackenzie, M., McDaid, D., Maxwell, M., Halliday, E. & Woodhouse, A. (2006). *Evaluation of the First Phase of Choose Life: The National Strategy and Action Plan to Prevent Suicide in Scotland*. Scottish Executive.

7 NHS Health Scotland (22 Aug. 2019). The art of conversation: A guide to talking, listening and reducing stigma surrounding suicide. Retrieved from http://www.healthscotland.com/documents/2842.aspx (accessed 1 Dec. 2020).

8 Distress Brief Intervention: https://www.dbi.scot/ (accessed 1 Dec. 2020).

9 Gilbert, P. (2010). *The Compassionate Mind*. Little, Brown Book Group.

10 Cleare, S., Gumley, A., O'Connor, R. C. (2019). Self-compassion, forgiveness, suicidal ideation and self-harm: A systematic review. *Clinical Psychology & Psychotherapy*. 26, 511–30.

11 Scottish Government (13 Jul. 2020). Adverse childhood experiences (ACEs). Retrieved from https://www.gov.scot/publications/adverse-childhood-experiences-aces/pages/trauma-informed-workforce (accessed 3 Dec. 2020).

# Chapter 13: Supporting Those Who Are Suicidal

1 Hawton, K., Saunders, K. E. A., & O'Connor, R. C. (2012). Self-harm and suicide in adolescents. *Lancet*, *379*, 2373–82.

2 Smith, D. M., Wang, S. B., Carter, M. L., Fox, K. R., & Hooley, J. M. (2020). Longitudinal predictors of self-injurious thoughts and behaviors in sexual and gender minority adolescents. *Journal of Abnormal Psychology*, *129*, 114–21.

3 Ferrey, A. E., Hughes, N. D., Simkin, S., Locock, L., Stewart, A., Kapur, N., Gunnell, D., & Hawton, K. (2016). The impact of self-harm by young people on parents and families: A qualitative study. *BMJ Open*, *6*, e009631.

4 Wasserman, D., Hoven, C. W., Wasserman, C., . . . & Carli, V. (2015). School-based suicide prevention programmes: The SEYLE cluster-randomised, controlled trial. *Lancet*, *385*(9977), 1536–44.

5 Researchers at the University of Oxford (26 Nov. 2015). Coping with self-harm: A guide for parents and carers. Retrieved from

https://www.psych.ox.ac.uk/news/new-guide-for-parents-who-are-coping-with-their-child2019s-self-harm-2018you-are-not-alone2019 (accessed 5 Dec. 2020).

6 Robinson, J., Teh, Z., Lamblin, M., Hill, N., La Sala, L., & Thorn, P. (2020). Globalization of the #chatsafe guidelines: Using social media for youth suicide prevention. *Early Intervention in Psychiatry*; chatsafe (n.d.). Tools and tips to help young people communicate safely online about suicide. Retrieved from https://www.orygen.org.au/chatsafe (accessed 27 Jan. 2020).

7 Luoma, J. B., Martin, C. E., & Pearson, J. L. (2002). Contact with mental health and primary care providers before suicide: A review of the evidence. *American Journal of Psychiatry, 159,* 909–16; Rhodes, A. E., Khan, S., Boyle, M. H., Tonmyr, L., Wekerle, C., Goodman, D., Bethell, J., Leslie, B., Lu, H., & Manion, I. (2013). Sex differences in suicides among children and youth: The potential impact of help-seeking behaviour. *Canadian Journal of Psychiatry, 58,* 274–82; National Confidential Inquiry into Suicide and Safety in Mental Health (Dec. 2019). Annual report 2019: England, Northern Ireland, Scotland and Wales. Retrieved from https://sites.manchester.ac.uk/ncish/reports/annual-report-2019-england-northern-ireland-scotland-and-wales (accessed 5 Jan. 2021).

8 Sayal, K., Yates, N., Spears, M., & Stallard, P. (2014). Service use in adolescents at risk of depression and self-harm: Prospective longitudinal study. *Social Psychiatry and Psychiatric Epidemiology, 49,* 1231–40.

9 Quinlivan, L., Cooper, J., Meehan, D., Longson, D., Potokar, J., Hulme, T., Marsden, J., Brand, F., Lange, K., Riseborough, E., Page, L., Metcalfe, C., Davies, L., O'Connor, R., Hawton, K., Gunnell, D., & Kapur, N. (2017). Predictive accuracy of risk scales following self-harm: Multicentre, prospective cohort study. *British Journal of Psychiatry, 210,* 429–36.

10 Bellairs-Walsh, I., Perry, Y., Krysinska, K., Byrne, S. J., Boland, A., Michail, M., Lamblin, M., Gibson, K. L., Lin, A., Li, T. Y., Hetrick, S., & Robinson, J. (2020). Best practice when working with suicidal behaviour and self-harm in primary care: A qualitative exploration of young people's perspectives. *BMJ Open, 10,* e038855.

11 McClelland, H., Evans, J., Nowland, R., Ferguson, E., & O'Connor, R. C. (2020). Loneliness as a predictor of suicidal ideation and behaviour: A systematic review and meta-analysis of prospective studies. *Journal of Affective Disorders, 274,* 880–96.

## Chapter 14: Surviving the Aftermath of Suicide

1 McDonnell, S., Hunt, I. M., Flynn, S., Smith, S., McGale, B., & Shaw, J. (2020). From grief to hope: The collective voice of those bereaved or affected by suicide. Suicide Bereavement UK. Retrievedfromhttps://suicidebereavementuk.com/the-national-suicide-bereavement-report-2020 (accessed 12 Dec. 2020).

2 Irons, A. (10 Sep. 2019). Twitter. Retrieved from https://twitter.com/AmyJIrons/status/1171460355798601731 (accessed 3 Feb. 2021).

3 Wertheimer, A. (2013). *A Special Scar.* Routledge; Fine, C. (2002). *No Time to Say Goodbye: Surviving the Suicide of a Loved One.* Bantam Doubleday Dell Publishing Group: Lukas, C., & Seiden, H.M. (2007). *Silent Grief: Living in the Wake of Suicide.* Jessica Kingsley Pub.

4 Support After Suicide Partnership (Sep. 2015). Help is at hand. Retrieved from https://supportaftersuicide.org.uk/resource/help-is-at-hand (accessed 13 Dec. 2020).

5 Sands, D. C. (2010). *Red Chocolate Elephants: For Children Bereaved By Suicide.* Karridale Pty Ltd.

6  Andriessen, K., Krysinska, K., Hill, N., Reifels, L., Robinson, J., Reavley, N., & Pirkis, J. (2019). Effectiveness of interventions for people bereaved through suicide: A systematic review of controlled studies of grief, psychosocial and suicide-related outcomes. *BMC Psychiatry*, *19*, 49.

7  Pitman, A., Osborn, D., King, M., & Erlangsen, A. (2014). Effects of suicide bereavement on mental health and suicide risk. *Lancet Psychiatry*, *1*, 86–94.

8  Sandford, D. M., Kirtley, O. J., Thwaites, R., & O'Connor, R. C. (2020). The impact on mental health practitioners of the death of a patient by suicide: A systematic review. *Clinical Psychology & Psychotherapy*.

9  These interviews were conducted as part of David Sandford's PhD research at University of Glasgow.

10 Department of Psychiatry, University of Oxford (11 Aug. 2020). New resource for psychiatrists: Patient suicide. Retrieved from https://www.psych.ox.ac.uk/news/new-resource-for-psychiatrists-patient-suicide (accessed 27 Jan. 2021).

# Index